FULLY ALIVE

DISCOVERING GOD'S HEART AND DESIGN FOR OUR HEALTH

DERYL W. DUER

PRAISE FOR *FULLY ALIVE*

"Deryl Duer has written a personal, inspirational, and challenging book showing the relationship between exercise, eating right, and biblical teaching. I knew Deryl when he was at his heaviest and unhealthiest, and it has been encouraging for me to watch his transformation, as well as his growing ministry in this pivotal area. I encourage you to ingest, digest, and act on his wisdom."

> —Kendell Easley, University Professor of Biblical Studies,
> Union University (Tennessee)

"I am the Sarah that you'll read about in this book. I have loved the Lord for many years, with all of my heart and mind but had never been taught about loving Him with all of my body. God began stirring in my heart this need to find out what His Word said about how to eat and care for my body. He led me to Deryl. What Deryl did for me over several months he has now done for you through this amazing book. I no longer see how I can sincerely love the Lord and willingly ignore the fact that He absolutely has a "best" for me in this area and that I was bought and paid for and that it is my responsibility, no, my privilege, to willingly bring this part of who I am under submission to Him. Why? Because it is His good pleasure that I live fully alive. Open your heart, read this with a willingness to learn, and the victory will be yours. I journey with you. It is indeed, war."

> —Sarah Musick, Christ-follower, wife, mother of 6 (with 7
> on the way), and worship leader

"For nearly a decade, I have enjoyed building a friendship with Deryl and Tracy that now can be described more as family. Being given the honor to mentor with Deryl as he worked this year to complete this God inspired mission, has more than blessed me personally. I have grown in my understanding of how every aspect of our lives is so important to God. I have learned to respect and love how He made me so that I can serve His purpose for my life reading through the chapters of this book. I encourage you to be prepared for your heart to receive the message God has for you as you take the journey to read Fully Alive. You will discover God's heart and design for your health!"

> —Denise Needham, CSO (Chief Strategy Officer),
> SurveyMe, Newport Beach, California

"Through his irrefutable testimony, Deryl exhorts us to commit to life fully. To be "All In." His honest, direct challenges are not formed in a bubble with a Bible, but with a life that contains tragedy and triumph. The Bible informs his experiences, giving meaning to his life, and in turn, to our lives. Our culture has grown weary of soft-spoken half-truths that make us feel better about our choices. Deryl's bold statements, backed with science and spirituality, lead us to authentic evaluation of our life now and how it could be in the future. Whether you consider yourself a health nut or a couch potato, this book will take you deeper in your understanding of complete health. Just as in the exhilarating conclusion of The Chronicles of Narnia, Deryl calls to us, "Come further up! Come further in!" Read this and gain a renewed desire to be Fully Alive!"

   —Jocelynn Bailey, Social Media and Communications
    Consultant

"Deryl has a passion to glorify the Lord in every aspect—and especially by being a steward of the temple that God has given him. In his book, he tells the story of his own dramatic 100-pound weight loss and transformation, encouraging others to be able to make the changes, too—and not out of vanity or as an idol, but as a tool to glorify the Maker of the heavens and the earth. He uses God's Word and his own personal experiences to remind you of the truth of the gift of obedience in all things to Christ. I encourage anyone to pick up this book to edify your spirit, encourage your mind, and motivate your body into submission to Christ. Every word of God proves true, he is a shield to those who take refuge in him. (Proverbs 30:5) May you be encouraged through the passion that God has given Deryl to proclaim this message!"

   —Keri Horning, CIHC, Founder, Energetic Wellness
    Coaching

FULLY ALIVE

DISCOVERING GOD'S HEART AND DESIGN FOR OUR HEALTH

DERYL W. DUER

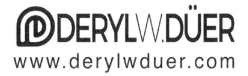

www.derylwduer.com

ISBN-13: 978-0692861707
ISBN-10: 069286170X
LCCN: 2017906625
BISCAC: Health & Fitness/Healthy Living

To my wife, Tracy—it is a blessing to share my life, love and purpose with you. This book would not be possible without your encouragement and support. And to our children, Reese, Sam, Gabe and Grace—thank you for your understanding and belief in your daddy's mission. Your growth in wisdom and stature and faith are a source of continual pride and joy.

ACKNOWLEDGMENTS

It has been said that writing a book is somewhat like birthing a child, and at times it has certainly felt like it. It has been a labor of love nearly a decade in the making and this material has been more lived than written. There are so many people I wish to thank who have inspired and encouraged me throughout this journey.

To Dana for being the first person to encourage me in this calling God has on my life and for giving me the first platform to teach. Words cannot express my gratitude. I look forward to seeing you again at the Master's table.

To Denise, for your guidance throughout the writing of this material, I could not have done this without you. Thank you for believing in this ministry and in me.

To our small group, friends and pastors at the Journey Fellowship campus of Oak Hills Church, thank you for supporting this vision and being my editors, readers and examples of what it looks like to walk with God.

To the staff at the Institute for Integrative Nutrition (IIN) and the "Write Your Dream Book" course, thank you for your passion for health and for giving me both the knowledge and support for writing, and a deadline to get it done.

To my family, whose love and support have never waivered through all of the ups and downs of life.

To Dad, for giving me kick in the pants I needed to take control of my health. Thank you. I am so grateful that God brought you back into my life.

To Mom, thank you for being a "nutrition nut" long before it was cool. I finally learned. Thank you for telling me I could do anything I set my mind to.

To my Lord and Savior, Jesus Christ, for the mighty power that You have displayed throughout my life. Thank You for Your grace and mercy, without which I would be lost. Thank you for creating and choosing me for such a time as this.

CONTENTS

INTRODUCTION

The glory of God is man fully alive.[1]
—SAINT IRENAEUS

"You missed my heart…"

Tears welled up in my eyes as I heard the voice of God speak those words to my spirit. It was a cool autumn morning and I was having my daily time alone with God on the back porch of our house in New Braunfels, Texas. I was reading John Eldredge's amazing book, *Waking the Dead*, and the quote from Saint Irenaeus leapt off the page at me—"The glory of God is man fully alive." God's voice immediately spoke to me, "Fully Alive! That's your title. There is your theme."

For nine years I had been writing and teaching God's principles for health and fitness that are found throughout the Bible. I had led weekly Bible studies, delivered sermons, blogged, and even led a weekend conference on the subject. Ever since my own 100-pound weight loss and health transformation, God had given me a passion to discover and teach what He has to say about taking care of our bodies.

You see, I was in seminary when I was at my heaviest weight and the unhealthiest point in my life. The years of intense study to finish my undergrad and start seminary, and the "sympathy weight" I gained along with my wife, Tracy, when she was pregnant with our first two children, had taken its toll. At the time, I just didn't know better. I didn't know what I was missing out on. I didn't know those were just excuses. My transformation had shown me how much better life was when I was healthy versus unhealthy.

That's when God started taking me back to His Word and showing me that it truly contains all of the advice we need for life. I was sharing my passion and what I was writing with my pastor at the time, Dana Key. Dana had been one of my heroes since I was a teenager. He was a pioneer of Christian rock music and half of Degarmo & Key, one of the biggest Christian bands of the 80's and early 90's. Dana was the first person to really suggest that God had set me apart for this ministry. He was also the first to warn me "as one pioneer to another" that the message God was giving me would not always be popular. He told me not to get discouraged when I experienced resistance from within the Church.

I started teaching these principles at our church, The Love of Christ Church, in Memphis, Tennessee. From the beginning I struggled with what to call it. Originally it was *Body by God*, then *Your Body is a Temple*, then *Fit4Glory*. None of those ever felt right. I never had a peace about them. Something was missing.

Enter the voice of God speaking to me in my quiet time that morning. Not only did He show me what I needed to call my study, but He also told me why. What I heard in my spirit that morning was this: "Fully Alive! That's your title. There is your theme. Everything you have written and taught the last nine years is correct. Your body is Mine. You are to glorify Me in it. I do care about what you eat and drink. I do care whether or not you are active. I do care about your health. All of those things are important, but you missed My heart."

That's when the tears welled up. Deep in my heart I knew it was the voice of God because I knew it was true. How had I missed that? After all of the amazing books on health and nutrition and fitness I had read, many of them written by Christians, how had I missed this?

God offers us *life*. Jesus says in John 10:10, "I have come that they may have life, and have it to the full" (John 10:10 NIV). Not some "pie-in-the-sky" dream, not just life in eternity, but a fully-abundant life right here, right now.

Is that what you're experiencing? Do you feel **fully** alive? I certainly didn't when I was overweight and had high blood pressure, pre-diabetes and high LDL cholesterol. Like most people, I was living a life I was comfortable with simply because I didn't know any different.

Most of us easily understand that Jesus came to give us eternal life, but it is not always as clear that eternal life begins *now*. The word *eternal* means "perpetual or everlasting," not "future." It's so much more than that. Luke 18:30 says that when we give our lives to Christ, we will be rewarded many times over "in this age, and in the age to come eternal life." When we are told that God's gift is eternal life, it means that it is ours forever. In other words, we can never lose it. As Oswald Chambers said, "I am not being saved—I am saved. Salvation is as eternal as God's throne, but I must put to work or use what God has placed within me."[2] The offer of life starts now. We must take care of all God has entrusted to us.

But what does this have to do with our health and fitness? There seems to be this sort of unspoken belief in the church that to concern ourselves with our bodies and fitness is, at best, a vain pursuit. About a week after my conversation with God about this book, a very dear friend named Sarah reached out to me. She said that God was prompting her to talk with me about her desire to be healthier. She said that she had always felt that working out and pursuing physical fitness were a form of idolatry—which, certainly they can be. But, she said, "I don't have any energy. I'm always tired. This can't be how we're meant to feel. I just want to be *fully alive.*"

I love Sarah's heart for God. She is completely in love with her Savior and God. She really wants to understand for herself whether or not God actually cares about her body and the effort required to keep it healthy and fit. Over the next couple of hours, we had a wonderful conversation exploring God's Word together, talking about the real world consequences of ignoring our health and the myriad of benefits that result from seeking to glorify God in our bodies. God began to reveal His heart to Sarah, and we all came away from that conversation encouraged.

Now, I invite you into that conversation.

Ask God to open the eyes of your heart to see His heart. I believe that our bodies are a gift from God. I believe it is His desire for us to be healthy and vibrant and strong so we can better serve Him. I believe it is His desire for us to bring every aspect of our being under His authority so that we can be *fully alive* in Him. That was Paul's prayer for us: "Now may the God of peace himself sanctify you completely, and may your whole spirit and soul and body be kept blameless at the coming of our Lord Jesus Christ" (1 Thessalonians 5:23 ESV).

Our spirit, soul and body are linked. If one suffers, the others also suffer. "All for one and one for all," as the saying goes. Being fully alive—living the life that God intended for us—requires being complete in Him. It means being as healthy and fit as we can be.

He's not asking for us to be athletes or models, but He does demand our best—our very best.

Are you ready to be fully alive?

SOLI DEO GLORIA (Glory to God Alone)

CHAPTER 1

WE ARE AT WAR

The thief comes only to steal and kill and destroy;
I have come that they may have life, and have it to the full.
—JESUS (JOHN 10:10 NIV)

Open war is upon you whether you would risk it or not.[1]
—ARAGORN (THE LORD OF THE RINGS:
THE TWO TOWERS)

I love *The Lord of the Rings*! Written by J.R.R. Tolkien, it is one of the greatest epic stories ever put to paper. Spread across three books, the adventure conveys so many deep truths about the nature of life and the struggles we all face. If you have no idea what I am talking about, I recommend you read the series—or at least see Peter Jackson's film adaptations.

In the second movie, *The Two Towers,* a dialogue takes place that many in the Church have quoted, especially as it relates to spiritual warfare. Théoden, king of the horse warriors of Rohan, is reluctant to go to battle. He is afraid, and rightfully so. A vast and overwhelming army of exceptionally vicious and powerful creatures called Uruk-hai is marching toward them, destroying everything in their path.

Aragorn, a main protagonist in the story and leader of the Fellowship of the Ring, tells Théoden, "It is an army bred for a single purpose: to destroy the world of men." Yet Théoden will not commit to battle. He is hesitant to accept the risk of what he knows it will cost.

"I will not risk open war," he balks.

Into his fear, Aragorn speaks truth: "Open war is upon you whether you would risk it or not."[2]

Tolkien's words through Aragorn hit the nail squarely on the head. Certainly, we can choose which battles we will fight, but the underlying fact is we were born into a world at war. Whether we like it, or not, there it is. We are at war—and we are losing too many of the battles badly. We lose them because, like Théoden, we hesitate to enter the battle, to fight for the life Jesus promised us.

Freedom is never free. We must fight for it.

Yes, Jesus promised us life, but He first warned us about a very real enemy who is waging war against us. He told us that our enemy is a thief whose sole intent is to steal and kill and destroy every aspect of our being. He has set himself and his armies against the life that Christ offers. The last thing our enemy wants is for us to be fully alive. He fears it. He knows what you are capable of in Christ, and it terrifies him.

That is why Peter warned us, "Be alert and of sober mind." Why? Because "Your enemy the devil prowls around like a roaring lion looking for someone to devour" (1 Peter 5:8 NIV).

Are you catching what Peter was saying here? You have an enemy who is on the hunt. He is on the offensive, and he is determined to do you harm. He doesn't want to just wound you. He doesn't want to scratch you. He wants to *devour* you, to tear you limb from limb. His attacks are merciless and brutal and he's looking to take out any believer who is not paying attention.

There is no "if" here. Peter considered it a given. We *will* be attacked by the enemy. And while those attacks may be subtle or unseen, they are most certainly savage and cruel and aimed to inflict the most damage possible. So Peter sounded the alarm and encouraged us to, "Resist him, standing firm in the faith, because you know that the family of believers throughout the world is undergoing the same kind of sufferings" (v. 9 NIV). James, the brother of Jesus, likewise encouraged us, "Resist the devil, and he will flee from you" (James 4:7 NIV).

If we are going to have any hope of resisting this enemy, we are going to need strength greater than our own. Thanks be to God that we do! "Finally, be strong in the Lord and in the strength of His might. Put on the full armor of God, so that you will be able to stand firm against the schemes of the devil" (Ephesians 6:10–11 NASB). We are soldiers in His army. We fight in His strength, by His authority and we are protected by supernatural armor. But we must be prepared. We most know in the deepest places of our hearts the tremendously high stakes of this battle. Losing is not an option—we must win this war!

I think we all sort of "know" these things on a surface level—like we know that the Allies stormed the beaches of Normandy on June 6, 1944. But that seems distant and far away. We have seen the pictures and heard the stories, but it's not real to us. Unless you were there, unless you experienced it first hand, it's hard to really *know*.

We have grown far too comfortable. We don't fully believe there is a spiritual war raging all around us. We close our eyes, which is the same as being blind. I know this because I was once blind too.

MY STORY

I was nineteen years old in the summer of 1989. I had made it through my freshman year at Florida State University and was living with my godfather (we called him "Uncle Joe") in Valdosta, Georgia. I hadn't exactly applied myself in school and was sort of floundering. Uncle Joe had helped me find a job working in pool construction. He thought that maybe some good, hard manual labor would help me get back on track. On a hot Saturday that August, Uncle Joe called me into the living room and told me to sit down. "I found your father," he said.

Huh? Come again. *You found my dad?*

"Yes. I made a couple of calls. He's living in Nashville. He should be at work now. I wrote the number down by the phone in the kitchen. Do what you want with it."

My mind started reeling. I could hardly breathe. It had been more than 12 years since I had seen, spoken with or heard from my father. I wasn't even sure if he was still alive. Yet, almost every time I was in a crowd I looked around, wondering if my dad was there somewhere. There was a hole in my heart and life left there by my father's absence.

Uncle Joe believed I needed my dad back in my life and so he found him.

Now what. What do I say?

I picked up the phone and dialed the number. A voice on the other end answered, "This is Deryl Duer."

Pause. *Hi, Dad*

An even longer pause. His voice breaking, my dad, hoping against hope, asked, "Deryl?"

Yes.

I don't recall the details of the call after that. I know there were lots of questions and lots of tears. My dad asked where I was and if he could come see me. He dropped everything he was doing, hopped in his Honda Accord and drove the 475 miles from Nashville to Valdosta as fast as he could. I'm pretty sure the posted speed limit signs were just suggestions to him that day because six hours later he knocked on the door of Uncle Joe's house. I opened the door and for the first time in more than 12 years I was face to face with my father.

He wrapped his arms around me and held me in a bear hug, the kind only a father can give. He just held me as we both wept. Eventually, we made it inside the house and sat down to talk, joined by Uncle Joe and his family.

Nothing can replace the years I lost with my father. I have to tell you though that this felt good. It was the beginning of our reconciliation and restoration as father and son. We got a second chance.

Now, I tell you that story to tell you this one:

Seventeen years later in August 2006, I was visiting my dad in Nashville along with my wife, Tracy, and our two oldest kids, Reese who was 2 and Sam who was 2 months. I was in the process of transferring to The Southern Baptist Theological Seminary, and we had driven up from Memphis to Louisville, Kentucky to visit the campus. On our way home, we decided to stop and spend some time with my dad. He pulled me aside at one point and with a concerned look on his face said, "Deryl, I'm worried about your health. You've gained a lot of weight the past couple of years."

You have to understand that I looked much different back then, much more like the Pillsbury Doughboy than Mr. Clean. I knew in my heart he was correct, but to be completely honest, I was more than a little offended. Maybe it was embarrassment. Maybe it was shame. Whatever it was, I didn't have time to really process because his next question pierced my heart even deeper and broke through all of my defenses. He asked, "Who's going to raise your boys when you're gone?"

Are you catching the irony of the moment? Do you understand how deeply that question rocked me to the core of my being? My father, the one who had abandoned me and left that gaping hole in my life, was warning me about the dangers of abandoning my own family—not temporarily, but for good.

When I got home to Memphis on Monday I made an appointment with my doctor to have a physical. He confirmed that my dad was right to be concerned. I was more than 100 pounds overweight and had high blood-pressure, high LDL cholesterol, and was borderline diabetic.

Because of what I had endured as a child, I promised myself I would be the best dad in the world and that I would never abandon my kids. I was determined to always be there for them. I decided that I would never be too tired to play with my kids. I envisioned running with them and wrestling with them and playing sports with them. But I wasn't keeping my promises.

Those days, I barely had the energy to walk up a flight of stairs. Ha! Who am I kidding? I got out of breath if I had to bend over and tie my shoes. My whole body was inflamed. You could see it in my skin, especially my face. And I felt it. I felt the pressure: the aches and the joints that hurt. My skin that just felt "tight." The inability to catch my breath at times. I wrestled with the fear that I was having a heart attack every time I got heartburn.

Do you know what I'm talking about?

I pray you don't. But I'm guessing you do—or that you love someone who does.

Here I was running the risk of losing my family every day. My choices were robbing me. I couldn't fully enjoy the days I did have with them. Ironically, it took my dad's warning that my future with them was in jeopardy to wake me up.

I put the emphasis on "my choices" because it's true. Motivational speaker Zig Ziglar used to say, "I have never accidentally eaten anything." That was me. I chose what I ate, when I ate, and how much I ate. I chose to be sedentary instead of investing time to exercise. As a result, I was slowly killing myself and significantly lowering my quality of life.

God gives us one body and one life to live, and I was abusing both of His gifts. So, I made the decision to do something about my health. I knew it was time to take action. I wasn't going to "try." I wasn't going to "see if it worked for me." No, I was going to *do it*! The Bible tells us, "I can do all things through him who gives me strength" (Philippians 4:13 NIV).

The first and most important aspect of creating any kind of lasting improvement in your life is simply faith. So, I took God at His Word.

That first day at the doctor's office, he wanted to put me on medications immediately to control my symptoms. However, I knew in my gut that pharmaceuticals were not the answer. I didn't want to treat the symptoms. I wanted to treat the underlying cause. Weeds must be pulled out by the roots. Simply cutting them doesn't work.

I also knew that if I started down that road it was a slippery slope to a life I did not want. I begged him for a chance to change my lifestyle. He gave me six weeks.

I started with an at-home six-week DVD workout program called Slim in 6˚ that my wife, Tracy, had ordered from an infomercial two years earlier. That's actually a funny story. A couple of weeks after Reese was born, Tracy was in the rocking chair nursing him and watching TV. I was headed out the door to go to church where I was an intern in the college ministry. She had been watching the infomercial and said she wanted to order it. She was looking for a way to get back into shape after pregnancy and the infomercial inspired her. I laughed and said something along the lines of nobody being able to get those results that fast, much less from an at-home workout. Maybe it was possible if you spent hours a day at a gym... But who was I to tell her no.

Tracy was working as a registered nurse, and I was working as an intern at our church. When the program came in she did it for a couple of days, but then she went back to work and got busy. And I wasn't being all that supportive as her husband—perhaps because I was nowhere close to where I needed to be with my fitness. Misery loves company, or so they say. So, on the shelf it went to be forgotten... until two years later.

I don't believe it's a coincidence that my doctor gave me six weeks to show improvements. We had a six-week program sitting at home on a shelf that guaranteed results. Even if I wasn't necessarily convinced, I had nothing to lose and was determined that nothing was going to stand in my way. Although I have to confess I didn't tell Tracy I was using it. We were on opposite schedules so I could do it while she was at work in the mornings and I had Reese and Sam down for naps. But I went all in, including making major changes to my diet in order to break my addiction to sugar and bad foods. I lost 27 pounds in those six weeks and lowered my blood pressure, cholesterol and blood sugar all to within normal ranges. When I went back for my six-week check-up, my doctor was completely flabbergasted! I was the first patient he had who had ever made such a dramatic change. In fact, he looked at the nurse and with a break in his voice said, "Whatever he paid today, refund it. I didn't do this, he did. I can't charge him for that."

A few weeks later, we were back at my dad's for Thanksgiving. I was down nearly 50 pounds from our visit three months earlier. When my brother, Zach, asked me what I was doing to lose weight so fast, I told him about my dietary changes and the at-home workout program. That was the first time I admitted to anyone I was using the program I had scoffed at. Tracy overheard our conversation and laughed. "You told me you were running," she said. That was true, I had run some, I just neglected to mention the part about using her DVDs. I had been through the program twice at that point and was looking for something new. That's when I found another at-home workout program called P90X®. It was time to take my fitness to the next level, so that was my Christmas gift to myself. I started my first round on January 1, 2007. I was excited and nervous at the same time—excited for what I dared to believe was possible and nervous because I knew it was going to be hard—really hard. I put the first DVD in for Chest & Back and heard Tony Horton say, "Don't say 'I can't,' say 'I presently struggle with.'" I did.

In all, I lost more than 100 pounds in just over seven months and was in the best shape of my life at 37 years old. But what I gained was even more powerful than all the weight I had lost. I gained a whole new life that I didn't even realize was possible. I didn't just get healthy. I created a new life for my family and me. It was only then that I began to understand how our health and fitness impacts every area of our life—for better or worse.

I am absolutely *committed* to being the best husband and father I can be. Even more important, I'm determined to glorify God with everything that I am and every aspect of my being, including my body. When I went back for my physical a year later, my doctor told me that if I had not changed my lifestyle there was a very good chance that I would have been dead by 45—and that my first warning sign may have been the heart attack that killed me. Instead, he said, I probably added 30-40 good years to my life! Maybe more.

That means I got a second chance with my family! I have more time to spend with my beautiful wife and now four amazing children. I got a second chance to be the person God made me to be and to *do* what he put me on earth to do. Fun side note—I was also a featured story in the P90X infomercial.

Which brings up another interesting thing that happened through that process. Our friends and family began to notice the changes in me and started asking me what I was doing. They began to ask for help. Of course I wanted to help, so I shared with them what was working for me. I encouraged them to start working out and helped them pick out a program based on their needs and likes. I also offered to help them with their meal plans and shared tricks I had learned along the way to save time and money and still eat healthy. As I studied verses that talk about glorifying God in our bodies (like 1 Corinthians 6:19-20), I began to realize that God has a *lot* to say about health.

Despite being raised in church and attending seminary, I couldn't recall a single time I had heard anyone talk about these things. So, I began to research and write and share with others what God was revealing to me through His Word. At this point, it wasn't a career, it was just a passion. I simply did it because I genuinely wanted to help people. But as T.D. Jakes said, "If you can't figure out your purpose, figure out your passion. For your passion will lead you right into your purpose."[3] Little did I know at the time that I was taking the first steps into a new life and career path.

Not long after this, I had the conversation with Dana when he encouraged me to pursue this as a ministry. Having a man of God I had admired for so many years speak a vision over me regarding what God was going to do was a turning point in my life. I began to read books about health and nutrition and exercise. I became a Certified Personal Trainer and Certified Turbo Kick˚, Insanity˚ and P90X˚ Instructor. I became a

Health Coach through the Institute for Integrative Nutrition. For the [?] my life I will continue my education in health and helping others because this is my passion.

I have a business and ministry that I *love* where I have the unspeakable privilege of helping others achieve their goals and live a healthy, fulfilling life. I get to help them live the kind of life God intended. To help them become fully alive.

LIFE OR DEATH

I call heaven and earth to witness against you today, that I have set before you life and death, blessing and curse. Therefore choose life, that you and your offspring may live.
—GOD (Deuteronomy 30:19 ESV)

I believe that God brings us through trials so we can help others. As Paul said, "Praise be to the God and Father of our Lord Jesus Christ, the Father of compassion and the God of all comfort, who comforts us in all our troubles, so that we can comfort those in any trouble with the comfort we ourselves receive from God" (2 Corinthians 1:3–4 NIV).

God has used my story to inspire others to make positive changes and to adopt a healthier, God-honoring lifestyle. This adventure is all about understanding that our physical bodies matter to God, that they are a precious gift, and that we will one day answer to Him for what we did with them. Put another way, it's about the choices we make.

Life is full of choices. Each and every choice you make has a consequence, either good or bad. And while we are free to choose our actions, we are not free to choose the consequences of those actions. Consequences are pre-determined by laws and principles ordained by God. Paul warns us in Galatians: "Do not be deceived: God is not mocked, for whatever one sows, that will he also reap" (Gal 6:7 ESV).

This is an absolute and universal truth. There are no exceptions. It applies to every area of life. It will either work for you or against you. Paul goes on to say: "Those who live only to satisfy their own sinful nature will harvest decay and death from that sinful nature. But those who live to please the Spirit will harvest everlasting life from the Spirit." (Gal 6:8 NLT)

It seems like an obvious choice, right? I mean, who would choose decay and death over eternal life? The Bible says that we are new creations in Christ (2 Corinthians 5:17) and yet we still struggle with our old sin nature. We believe the Devil's lie when he says we can break God's laws and get away with it. We rationalize; we creatively justify our rebellious behavior;

we convince ourselves that we won't face any real consequences. We have this strange idea that doing whatever we feel like is freedom. It never seems to work out that way though.

What we find is that the more we pursue our idea of freedom, the more we discover it is a trap. Freedom does not mean the absence of moral constraints or absolutes. Remember that part about not being free to choose the consequences of our actions? Let's take the law of gravity as an example.

Suppose you go skydiving and at 10,000 feet you announce to the rest of the group, "I'm not using a parachute this time. I want freedom!" The fact is that you are constrained by a greater law than your idea of freedom—the law of gravity. If you choose the "constraint" of the parachute, you save your life and enjoy the positive consequence that comes with the freedom and exhilaration of the experience. If not, you'll suffer the negative consequences of severe injury and, probably, death.

God's laws act the same way: they restrain us, but they are absolutely necessary to enjoy the exhilaration of real freedom. Likewise, our bodies are subject to certain "laws" when it comes to nutrition, exercise, and so forth. Obey those laws, and you experience the positive consequences of feeling better, living longer, and enjoying a more abundant life. Disregard them and you have nobody but yourself to blame for the negative consequences of disease, discomfort and early death.

We are each responsible for our lives because we are responsible for our choices. Your challenge is to own up to your responsibility for your current state of health. As Darren Hardy said in his book, *The Compound Effect*:

> From this day forward, choose to be 100 percent responsible for your life. Eliminate all of your excuses. Embrace the fact that you are freed by your choices, as long as you assume personal responsibility for them. It's time to make the choice to take control.[4]

That day at my dad's house was my wake-up call to the health issues in my own life. It was the day I decided to own my responsibility for my health and take control. I thank God that my dad loved me enough to confront me with the truth, that he was "courageously forthright" as one of my mentors likes to say. I knew I had to make drastic changes. I was fortunate enough that I woke up when I did or my wake up call may have been the heart attack that killed me.

God had plans for me. I believe He has plans for you too. But we can no longer afford to ignore what is going on all around us. The United States is facing a massive health crisis that is tied to an obesity epidemic.

This situation is getting worse every year, despite the ever-increasing number of diets and gyms popping up. These are the facts:

- Adult obesity rates have more than doubled since 1980, while childhood obesity rates have more than tripled.[5] It is estimated that by 2030, 13 states will have adult obesity rates over 60 percent and all 50 states will have obesity rates over 44 percent.[6]
- Nearly 3/4 of American men and more than 60 percent of American women are overweight (Body Mass Index (BMI) of 25-30) or obese (BMI > 30)—the majority of them are obese. The result is millions of new cases of diabetes, coronary heart disease, strokes and other chronic illnesses.[7]
- Diabetes, coronary heart disease and other "lifestyle-based diseases" now kill more people than infectious disease worldwide.[8]
- One in two Americans suffer from "diabesity"—a term coined by Dr. Francine Kaufman to describe the spectrum of imbalance that ranges from mild insulin resistance to pre-diabetes to full-blown diabetes. The scariest part is that 90 percent of the people suffering from this very serious health condition don't even know it.[9]
- For the first time in history, this generation of children will live less healthful and shorter lives than their parents.[10]
- For the first time in history, as many people are suffering from the result of too much food as malnutrition. We see the commercials of people all over the world struggling from not having enough food to eat, or clean water to drink, while millions more people are struggling from the effects of excess calorie-dense, nutrient-poor foods and chemical laden beverages.[11]

According to a panel of national nutrition and health experts, obesity is "the single greatest threat to public health in this century"[12]— and the Church isn't immune. In fact, we appear to be part of the problem.

A 2006 study conducted by Purdue University Professor Ken Ferraro examined the relationship between religion and obesity.[13] The study found that fundamental Christians are more likely to be overweight or obese than the general public. We are, by far, the heaviest of all religious groups, led by Baptists at a 30 percent obesity rate, compared with Jews at 1 percent and Buddhists and Hindus at 0.7 percent. These findings prompted Ferraro, a professor of sociology who has studied religion and body weight since the early 1990s, to comment, "America is becoming known as a nation of gluttony and obesity, and churches are a feeding ground for this problem."

Ferraro is not alone in his findings. In 2007, *SBCLife*, the Journal of the Southern Baptist Convention, published an article entitled, "Obesity in the Body of Christ."

The article lamented:

> Unfortunately, our own statistics lend support to Ferraro's findings. . . . An Executive Summary Report of Wellness Center statistics for the 2005 convention showed that more than 75 percent of the 1,472 participants who completed the screening were found to be significantly overweight. Compare this to the national estimate that approximately 65 percent of adults are considered overweight, and you see a problem that the church must address.[14]

A 2011 study conducted by Northwestern University tracked 3,433 men and women for 18 years and found that young adults who attend church or a Bible study once a week are 50 percent more likely to be obese by middle age as their non-religious peers.[15] Matthew Feinstein, the study's lead investigator and a fourth-year student at Northwestern University Feinberg School of Medicine, suggested, "It's possible that getting together once a week and associating good works and happiness with eating unhealthy foods could lead to the development of habits that are associated with greater body weight and obesity." Feinstein also recognized that the church can play a significant role in reversing the trend of obesity. "Here's an opportunity for religious organizations to initiate programs to help their congregations live even longer," Feinstein said. "The organizations already have groups of people getting together and infrastructures in place that could be leveraged to initiate programs that prevent people from becoming obese and treat existing obesity."[16]

Likewise, the Pawtucket Heart Health Program found that people who attended church are more likely than non-church members to be 20 percent overweight and have higher cholesterol and blood pressure.[17] A 2001 Pulpit and Pew study of 2,500 clergy found that 76 percent were overweight or obese compared to 61 percent of the general population at the time of the study.[18]

There is no doubt that excess weight poses a very serious threat to our physical health, but it goes beyond even that. As unhealthy believers, we are greatly limiting our usefulness in kingdom work.

In a 2012 op-ed for FoxNews, Scott Stoll, M.D., observed, "The obesity epidemic in the church appears to be undermining the primary purpose of the church and its missions work by straining church budgets, decidedly absorbing money that would be spent on missions abroad, and consuming the time and energy of pastors and church members."[19]

Dr. Stoll went on to say, "The contemporary church culture has unwittingly contributed to the rise in overweight and obese parishioners. Today it is rare to hear a sermon preached on the stewardship of the physical body and even more rare on the vice of gluttony; it has become a secret and acceptable vice in the modern church."

Before I go any further, I also need to point out that this is not just about obesity. Most people understand that there is a relationship between being overweight and disease. What most people don't realize—and what has recently been discovered—is that being thin doesn't automatically mean you're not fat. You could be TOFI (Thin Outside, Fat Inside) or "skinny fat." That means that you have a higher ratio of visceral fat, the fat stored around your organs, and you are at as much risk of diabetes and heart disease as someone who is obese. According to a study published in 2012 in the Journal of the American Medical Association, one quarter of Type 2 Diabetics (21 percent) maintain a normal weight and yet have twice the mortality rate of obese diabetics.[20]

Enough is enough! These warnings should be a wake-up call to all of us, especially the Church. Scripture commands us to care for and heal the sick (Matthew 10:8). It is wrong that a lack of physical fitness is so common in our society that we view it as normal and healthy people are dismissed as "health nuts." The sad truth is that we have ignored the biblical mandate to glorify God in our bodies and are reaping the consequences of our sin.

As Dr. Stoll pointed out, odds are that you have never heard a sermon about the importance of taking care of our physical bodies—about the impact of our health and fitness on our ability to serve the Kingdom of God at all times and in every way—and yet the Bible is very clear on the subject. As Rick Warren said, "The Bible, and Scriptures, are literally filled with health advice—we just ignore it."[21]

We easily recognize the health risks of smoking, alcohol abuse, and sex outside of marriage. We understand that it is sinful to engage in these habits and encourage abstinence. We understand that whatever momentary pleasure may be derived from them, the negative consequences are simply not worth it. So what's the disconnect when it comes to our fitness?

Our quest is to search the Scriptures to see what God has to say about taking care of our bodies and to develop a biblical theology of health and fitness. From Genesis to Revelation we will see that God places very high value on our physical bodies. We'll discover that not only are our bodies important to God, but that He is also particularly concerned with what we do with our bodies. As Christians, anything that is important to God should be important to us. Whatever He places value on, we should also place value on. Things that are a priority for Him should be a priority for us. By God's grace, we will come away with a new appreciation of these amazing bodies He has given us and a commitment to glorify Him in them.

DANA'S LEGACY

I stood on the floor of an arena in Tampa, Florida, excitedly waiting for the concert to begin. I was a senior at Dr. Phillips High School in Orlando, Florida, and had driven down to the concert with some friends from church. The air was thick with anticipation. The lights went out and the unmistakable voice of Dana Key pierced the darkness.

No guitars. No keyboard. No drums. Just Dana soulfully belting out the chorus of *Casual Christian*:

I don't want to be, I don't want to be a casual Christian
I don't want to live, I don't want to live a lukewarm life
'Cause I want to light up the night with an everlasting light
I don't want to live a casual Christian life.[22]

It was a powerful kick off to an amazing concert. For those of you old enough to remember Christian rock legends Degarmo & Key, you recognize this powerful call to abandon mediocrity and live full on for Christ. If you knew Dana, you know that was the theme of his life. Dana loved Jesus! Correction, Dana loves Jesus and is singing right now before his King. I bet he has a new white guitar too—a heavenly Stratocaster.

My relationship with Dana began in 1985. *Commander Sozo & The Charge of The Light Brigade* was one of the very first Christian music cassettes I owned. I won it at youth group and was so proud of it. I soon bought their previous release, *Communication*. Music has always been a big part of my life, and I loved theirs. It got me through a very tough time.

Our youth group was going snow skiing that Spring Break. I woke up at 6:00 on Saturday morning, March 9, 1985, excited to get to the Second Baptist Church parking lot to meet the youth group for our long drive from Huntsville, Texas, to Santa Fe, New Mexico. As I walked down the hallway I could tell that the TV was on.

That's strange, I thought. *Dad shouldn't be home yet.*

My dad was a police officer with the Huntsville Police Department and worked the night shift. I should probably clarify this for you, since you remember me telling you that my biological dad was missing from my life for 12 years. This was Kevin Williams, my stepdad technically, although step-dad doesn't quite cut it. He married my mom when I was eight and from the beginning raised my brother, Zach, and me like we were his own. He even adopted us.

That's where the "W" comes from in my name: Deryl Williams Duer. I keep his name to honor the man who raised me and was a father to me— even though he didn't have to be. My sister, Laurie, was born in 1981. So on this spring morning of 1985, my family consisted of me at 15 years old, my brother Zach was 9, Laurie was 3 and my mom and Kevin.

On this particular day, I expected Kevin to be home to take me up to the church, but not for another hour or so. As I got near the end of the hall I could see he wasn't the one sitting on the couch. It was another officer that everyone called "Frosty."

That's strange. Maybe Frosty got in trouble at home and needed a place to crash.

Not that I had any reason to think that was true, it just seemed like the most "logical" explanation. As I cleared the end of the hall though, I could see that his wife was sitting on that side of the couch.

Okay, this is really strange.

I kept walking into the kitchen to get a glass of water. Frosty and his wife got up and followed me into the kitchen.

"Hi, Deryl. I'm Frosty," he said. "I work with your dad."

"I know," I replied.

"I don't know how else to tell you this," he continued. "Your dad's been shot. He's been taken to Houston. It doesn't look good."

And just like that, my world crumbled.

They managed to keep Kevin alive until his parents, my Nana and Gramps, could get back to Houston from their vacation in Hawaii. Gramps was Dr. Robert L. Williams, and he served as Chief of Psychiatry and Neurology in the USAF Surgeon General's Office. He was also a special advisor to several presidents and foreign heads of state. There were even stories of him advising President John F. Kennedy during the Cuban Missile Crisis.

Needless to say, Gramps was a big deal and had friends in high places, particularly in the medical community. He served as President of numerous medical societies both in Texas and around the country, and was a member of even more. At the time, he headed the Psychiatry department at Baylor College of Medicine in Houston. He was also a prolific writer and authored or co-authored numerous books and medical journal articles.

I tell you all of that to tell you that Gramps had pull. He knew people. He counted the best medical professionals in the world among his friends. So, when he got the news that Kevin had been shot, Gramps started making calls. But the most brilliant neurosurgeons in the world couldn't help his son—the man I called my dad. Kevin had been shot with a .22 rifle. The bullet entered his brain and had not been able to exit the skull, so it ricocheted around inside. The officers who first arrived on the scene had been able to get his heart going again, but he was brain dead before his body hit the ground.

For the second time in my life I had lost a dad. And although Kevin had given his life saving a woman from her homicidal estranged husband, it still felt like I'd been abandoned. I was proud of him, but I was also hurt and angry.

We had a memorial service on Monday, and my family decided that I needed to be with my youth group more than anything else. I needed the comfort and support of my friends and my youth pastor. I was entering a dark time in my life. I needed all the help I could get.

As I'm writing this, I'm listening to Degarmo & Key on iTunes. Inspiration, I guess. It brings back memories. You know how you can hear a song that you haven't heard in decades and you're immediately transported back to that time in your life? I still know all the words to all of the songs. And I almost forgot what an amazing guitar player Dana was. Yep, he's definitely playing a guitar in Heaven.

My point, though, is that these songs are ingrained in my mind and heart because they were my anthems at a time when my faith was all I had. They helped get me through those turbulent years.

I went to four Degarmo & Key concerts during high school and college. I got to meet Dana when I served as a prayer partner and counselor at a concert in Houston in 1991. I remember being impressed with how real he was and how much he really cared for people. His mission was to reach people for Christ through his music. I saw him pray with kids and lead them to Christ. He was the real deal. I wanted to be like him when I "grew up."

I really got to *know* Dana after Tracy and I had moved to Memphis in 1999. I was playing guitar with the worship team at Germantown Baptist Church, along with a singles Bible study called Metro. Dana was a member of the church at that time and leading the largest Sunday school class in the church. In 2002, Dana started The Love of Christ Church (TLC).

I told you . . . Dana loved Jesus!

When Tracy and I began attending TLC Church in early 2009, Dana invited us to meet with him because he wanted to get to know us. That's when I began to share my journey with him. He had known who I was as part of the Metro band, so he had seen me when I was at my heaviest. He was impressed with my transformation and asked about my story. Remember the conversation where Dana encouraged me by saying that God had set me apart for this ministry? This is when that happened.

I had the privilege over the next couple of years to meet with Dana on several occasions. I was invited to weekly prayer meetings. He became a mentor to me. As one of his biggest fans, that was so cool!

Then Dana asked me for help. He had been struggling with some health issues and knew he needed to get control of his health. He invited me to teach on Wednesday nights at church and take church members through what at that time was called "Your Body Is a Temple." I started working with Dana and his wife, Anita. They were making progress, but Dana was under a lot of stress and got off track for a bit. After church, Sunday, May 30, 2010, Dana told me he knew it was time to get back on track with his health and asked if I would help him again.

I was honored, of course. Dana and Eddie Degarmo had started playing together again and were scheduled to do a fundraising concert at the church in a couple of weeks. Things seemed to be looking up. A week later, we got the call that Dana suffered some kind of medical episode and we needed to get to the hospital as quickly as possible. It turned out to be a pulmonary embolism. We stood in the hospital waiting room with Dana's family and friends. We prayed, but it was too late. Dana was gone.

When we were allowed to go back into the hospital room to say our goodbyes, I wept. We all wept.

As I stood alone by Dana's bed, holding his hand, tears streaming down my face, I kept thinking *It's too late. I'm too late. This can't be happening. Not again.*

Twenty-five years earlier I had stood by Kevin's bed, holding his hand, overcome with grief—and regret. Just a few hours earlier I had watched him walk out the door to go to work. I was a typical 15-year-old boy, which means I was "pushing the envelope" with my dad. I had been testing his limits. I was alone on the couch, folding clothes to pack for the ski trip when a voice in my head said, "Tell him you love him." The words never made it out of my mouth, and Kevin walked out the door.

As I stood by his hospital bed the next day I couldn't say it enough. But it was too late. In my heart, I know he knew that I loved him, but I missed my last chance to tell him.

It was too late.

I missed my last opportunity to help Dana. I was too late. He was too late.

Those missed opportunities to serve the Kingdom of God are immeasurable.

I have a photo album on my phone of things that inspire me. One of them, the first one actually, is a picture of Dana and me. It was taken in Nashville at a coach training and workout I was hosting in October 2009. Dana and Jason Scheff (bass player and lead vocalist for the band Chicago) led a live jam session for our group workout. That was an awesome day!

I keep that photo as a reminder of *why* I do what I do. The world lost a great man when Dana passed. Anita lost her husband. Their children, Scottie, Andrew, and Eli, lost their father. His parents lost their son. His sisters, Jaime and JoLynn, lost their brother. I lost a friend and mentor, a man who had become like a father to me.

I think of all of the lives Dana still could have touched. When we experience unexpected losses like that, we say things to comfort each other like, "It was his time to go." That's what everyone said when Kevin died. That's what we all said when Dana died. But, I question that. It sounds spiritual, but I don't know.

Is God sovereign? Yes, absolutely!

Does he know all of our days? Yes.

Are they numbered? Yes. But…

Is it possible that our decisions affect the number of days we have? Yes.

We reap what we sow. If you play Russian roulette every day, you increase your risk of dying prematurely. If you play "Russian roulette" with your health, the same thing happens. God knows what decisions you will make and somehow they are factored in with His sovereignty. Don't ask me how that works. I have no clue. It's above my pay grade. All I know is that both truths are at work.

The picture of Dana reminds me of what is at stake. We are at war, and this *is* a life or death issue. Heart disease, which is what killed Dana, is at least 80 percent preventable with proper lifestyle changes. According to the American Heart Association, 614,348 Americans died from heart disease in 2014.[23] So, if it's 80 percent preventable, that means that more than 491,478 of the deaths in 2014 could have been prevented. It's actually probably higher than that.

And that's just heart disease. Type 2 Diabetes is just as deadly and is just as preventable. Odds are, you or someone you love will die from something that is preventable.

Yes, we will all die. That is not preventable. How and when we die, well, more often than not, that is determined by our choices. Where are your choices leading you? Will you lead a long and full life to the glory of God, or will you allow the thief to steal your life and rob the world of the gifts God gave you to share? God has set before you life and death.

Please—choose life.

CHAPTER 2

KNOW YOUR ENEMY

For we do not wrestle against flesh and blood, but against the rulers, against the authorities, against the cosmic powers over this present darkness, against the spiritual forces of evil in the heavenly places.
—THE APOSTLE PAUL (Ephesians 6:12 ESV)

The Church lives in a hostile world. Within and around her are enemies that not only could destroy her, but are meant to and will unless she resists force with yet greater force.[1]
—A.W. TOZER

If you know your enemy and know yourself, you need not fear the result of a hundred battles. If you know yourself but not the enemy, for every victory gained you will also suffer a defeat. If you know neither the enemy nor yourself, you will succumb in every battle.[2]
—SUN TZU, The Art of War

In the first of Peter Jackson's *The Lord of the Rings* trilogy, *The Fellowship of the Ring*, Frodo, the Hobbit and ring bearer, is on the run from the evil black riders. They are the Nazgûl, formerly great kings of men who are now servants of the dark lord, Sauron. Frodo is confronted by the Ranger, Strider (who turns out to be King Aragorn). Strider, who has been sent to help Frodo, asks him, "Are you frightened?" Frodo answers, "Yes." Strider replies, "Not nearly frightened enough. I know what hunts you."[3]

Do you know what hunts you?

Yes, at its core, this is a spiritual battle. Yes, there is a Devil and the demonic hosts—the spiritual forces of evil. But they have allies. They are rulers and authorities. Rulers and authorities over what? This present darkness. The world's system.

God has a plan for you and your health. God's plans are to "prosper you and not to harm you, plans to give you a future and a hope" (Jeremiah 29:11, NIV). But the enemy has plans for you too, and you won't like where they lead very much. While God offers a future and hope, the enemy promises pain and destruction.

So how do you recognize the enemy? Here's a pretty good general rule: Find out what "everybody else" is doing and do the opposite. Jesus said that the gate to life is narrow, and few people choose it. In contrast, the road to destruction is wide and heavily traveled (Matthew 7:13-14). He was talking about salvation, but the principle applies universally. If something looks like the easy way, it's probably a trap.

As I wrote that, I had this vision of General Akbar in *The Return of the Jedi* saying, "It's a trap." Don't trust the easy way. There are no shortcuts. Everything in life worth having or doing requires work—lots of it. Name me an exception. You can't, can you?

So, look at who's offering you shortcuts and the "easy" way. Chances are good that the enemy is behind it.

Are you beginning to see? If not, that's okay. I'm confident you will. I pray with the Apostle Paul that the eyes of your heart may be enlightened (Ephesians 1:18). Are you ready to open your eyes?

EYES TO SEE

On a dark and stormy night, in a dimly lit room in a decrepit building two men meet for the first time, although we later learn they have been searching for one another for most of their lives. The older of the two, a tall black man named Morpheus, is dressed from head to toe in black. He is wearing a leather trench coat and dark glasses that are held on to his face without the aid of side temples. It's a rather Goth look. We sense that he knows things—deep truths that escape most people.

The younger man, named Neo, has come to him because he is searching for something. On the table before him is a clear glass of water. Neo is clearly uneasy, but he has to know. Morpheus closes the door to the room leaving them alone. Thunder and lightning crash.

Morpheus senses Neo's discomfort. He tells Neo that he knows he is probably feeling a lot like Alice, tumbling down the rabbit hole. He knows because he was once in Neo's seat. Neo has heard rumors of something called the Matrix and this mysterious man called Morpheus.

Morpheus tells Neo that he knows why he has come. He knows that Neo is in search of something he can't explain, like a nagging thought that dances just out of reach. He is searching for the Matrix.

Morpheus tells Neo that the Matrix is the world that has been pulled over his eyes to blind him to the truth—the truth that we are slaves. It is a prison of ignorance designed to keep us complacent and apathetic—lukewarm. As with most things, we cannot be told what the Matrix is, we must see it for ourselves, and so Morpheus offers Neo a choice.

Morpheus leans forward and holds both hands out in front of him. In one is a blue pill, in the other a red one. He explains to Neo that if he takes the blue pill, the story will end and he will wake up in his bed thinking it was all a dream and go on believing whatever he wants to believe. But if Neo takes the red pill, he will stay in Wonderland and Morpheus will show him just how deep the rabbit hole goes.

Neo has been offered a choice. He can choose ignorance and go back to his "normal" life where truth is whatever is most convenient and nothing is ever questioned. Or he can have his eyes opened to see the truth, knowing that once he does he can never go back to his old life.

Neo chooses the red pill. He chooses truth.

What will you choose?

When it comes to health, we too are caught in a "matrix" of sorts. The world we think we see is not real. It's a lie that has been pulled over our eyes. We should not be surprised. This has been the strategy of our enemy from the beginning. The Fall occurred as the result of a wrong choice regarding food. God had supplied Adam and Eve with everything they needed for life, every kind of amazing food imaginable. There was only one rule, one thing that was forbidden. The fruit of one tree.

The serpent lied to Eve. He created doubt about God's provision and goodness. He sowed the seeds of confusion. He does the same thing today, only now it is through powerful allies who control the narrative. There are industries out there being used by the enemy to confuse you and to rob you of your health and your life. Are you able to open your eyes to see how deep the rabbit-hole goes?

THE FOOD INDUSTRY

It is estimated that Americans spent as much as $2.1 trillion on food in 2016.[4] Let me write that out for you so you see it—that's $2,100,000,000,000. Food is big business!! More than half of the money we spend on food goes to restaurants and fast-food establishments.[5] Sitting around the table together over a good home-cooked meal seems to only happen at holidays. But that's only part of the problem. Even when we do eat at home, more often than not, we are eating highly processed "convenience" foods. According to research, nearly 60 percent of calories and 90 percent of added sugar in the American diet come from "ultra-processed foods."[6] I'm having to resist the urge to open that one up right now, but I promise we will get to it.

It's not entirely our fault. Slick advertising designed to hit every possible trigger bombard us each day. And it's not just the pizza and burger and frosted sugar ads that should worry us. The health concerns that accompany rising obesity rates have prompted many food manufacturers to focus on key marketing terms, such as "low-fat," "whole grain," "gluten free,"—whatever the buzz word is at the moment—to promote their products. But when you turn the box over and study the ingredients you find that this is not food. This is a chemistry experiment. I've heard them referred to as "frankenfoods." I love that one. You see, for the food industry, mixed messages and confusion are good for business.

Author Michael Pollan has noted:

As a journalist I fully appreciate the value of widespread public confusion: We're in the explanation business, and if the answers to the questions we explore got too simple, we'd be out of work. Indeed, I had a deeply unsettling moment when, after spending a couple years researching nutrition for my last book, *In Defense of Food*, I realized that the answer to the supposedly incredibly complicated question of what we should eat wasn't so complicated after all, and in fact could be boiled down to just seven words: *Eat food. Not too much. Mostly plants.*[7]

That's it in a nutshell. God's plan to feed our bodies summed up in seven simple words. God's food is pure. It is simple. It is alive. God's food contains *no* artificial colors and flavors. It has no pesticides or preservatives. You won't find any high-fructose corn syrup, growth hormones, or antibiotics. Genetically modified organisms (GMO's) are nowhere to be found. God knew what He was doing when he created plants for food—they are perfect in their natural form.

Oh, and it just so happens that modern nutrition science, at least what's not funded by a highly-invested entity, backs this up. And therein lies the problem—the bottom line.

Economics drives the food industry—not your health. In many cases, leaders in the food industry don't care about you or your family. They care about their bottom line. At best, they are pawns of our spiritual enemy. Some of them are even his allies; and, until you come to terms with this and begin to understand the depths to which they go to confuse and enslave you, you're going to have a hard time fighting back.

The battle begins in your mind. The food industry spends billions of dollars a year on ads that are calculated to make us eat more and more of the worst possible food. And by "ads," I don't just mean commercials on TV or full-color spreads in magazines. Those boxes and cans of food lined up at the grocery store are ads too. Broccoli doesn't have a slick ad campaign. There is no fancy packaging. It doesn't need it. God packaged it perfectly. But God is not driven by profit. He is our Father. He is motivated by love.

The food industry, on the other hand, is driven by profit. I get that. It's not a totally bad thing in and of itself. They have to make money to stay in business—though we would be much better off if some of them *did* go out of business. You see, generally speaking, there is an inverse relationship between nutritional value and financial profit when it comes to food. The more you process any food, the more profitable it becomes. But the more you process it, the less nutritional value it retains.

That's why we see things like enriched flour. The manufacturers try to cram nutrients they processed out back in, but it doesn't work. What we end up with is a far cry from what God gave us. Packaged and processed food companies spare no expense to push more of their products on their target market. Did you know that more than 90 percent of their product sales are made to less than 10 percent of their customers and that in the case of processed foods that 10 percent consists primarily of people who weigh more than 200 pounds and earn less than $35,000 a year?[8] That's because one of the laws of marketing is that it's easier to sell more product to an existing customer than to cultivate a new one. Where it becomes tragic is the case of processed foods. For processed food companies, including fast-food companies, that all-important 10 percent consists largely of people who are significantly overweight and, in many cases, living on lower incomes.

In his book, *The New Wellness Revolution*, economist Paul Zane Pilzer observed:

> No expense is spared to hit every psychological button that matters to the target market. . . . Like a deer caught in the scope of a hunter at close range, the target never has a chance. At times, the ruthlessness of the process troubles the consciences of the $200,000-per-year marketing executives in charge of it. Some actually refuse to attend their own focus groups. Rather than confront their future victims in person, they prefer to review transcripts in the safety of their offices.[9]

Are you shocked? Did you know that? I didn't know that. I mean, at a certain level I knew I was being sold a bill of goods, but I didn't realize it was that bad. In fact, I probably knew that a little better than most. My father was a commercial photographer in Nashville and some of his biggest accounts were restaurants—everything from fast-food places to nice sit-down restaurants.

When these businesses would come in to the studio to do a shoot, they brought an army with them—marketing executives, cooks, food stylists. Let's say the shot was a plate of chicken strips and French fries. They would bring cases of each and fry several baskets just to get the perfect specimens. Then the food stylists went to work with their tools placing and manipulating the plate until it was picture perfect—literally. It would take an entire day to get maybe four shots in.

Now you know why what you order never quite looks like what's on the menu.

The first weapon of the enemy is to entice you. But wait—it actually gets worse. These companies also have teams of scientists whose job is to create these "frankenfoods." They create processed foods that are irresistibly appealing and addictive. That's how they really get their hooks into you. These foods have been twisted and altered in such a way that the manufacturers know you can't eat just one. Numerous books and documentaries have begun exposing this scandal, and it's not just coming from a "fringe" element. We are seeing more and more health professionals speaking out as they learn the truth. In his book, *The Blood Sugar Solution,* Dr. Mark Hyman said:

> Food scientists focus on creating foods that maximally trigger the "bliss point," that addictive reward pathway in the brain that keeps you coming back for more. . . . Big Food spends millions on food science and hires "craving experts" to ensure that its customers will become addicted to deviously developed drugs, all of which are hidden in cleverly disguised delivery vehicles for sugar, fat, and salt. Think heroin lollipops.[10]

It sounds like an exaggeration, but it's not. Look around you. Look in the mirror. You see the effects of the enemy's attacks everywhere. This is no accident—it is a deliberate calculation designed to enslave us. And what about our government? Shouldn't they be protecting us from this kind of deception? Isn't that the job of the FDA?

Nope.

In fact, the FDA isn't even on your side. It's on the side of industry. And that's not just my opinion. It's a fact.[11] Even the food guidelines are wrong.

They are bought and paid for. Dr. Walter C. Willet, chairman of the Department of Nutrition at the Harvard School of Public Health and professor of medicine at Harvard Medical School, said this:

> The thing to keep in mind about the Pyramid is that it comes from the arm of the federal government responsible for promoting American agriculture. It doesn't come from agencies established to monitor and protect our health, . . . And there's the root of the problem—what's good for agricultural interests isn't necessarily good for the people who eat their products.[12]

Fortunately, many are beginning to wake up and understand that we must take responsibility for ourselves—and our families. We need to become our own health advocates. We are beginning to demand changes. People are voting with their wallets as it were. If you want the industry to change, you have to give them a reason, and they only respond to profits.

THE "HEALTHCARE" SYSTEM

The question of getting more people access to health care has been one of the most heated political debates of the past several decades, but it seems to have reached new heights since the introduction of the Patient Protection and Affordable Care Act, better known as Obamacare. We could argue back and forth all day about this law from a political perspective, but we would still miss the most important point. Ultimately it will fail—not because it was right or wrong, but because it answered the wrong question.

A better question, the right question, is how can we create a health care system that actually helps people be healthier. That might seem like a novel idea, but that's not what we have in the United States. We have what Dr. Andrew Weil calls "a disease-management system—one that depends on ruinously expensive drugs and surgeries that treat health conditions after they manifest rather than giving our citizens simple diet, lifestyle and therapeutic tools to keep them healthy."[13]

You see the harsh reality is that Americans spend far more per capita on healthcare than any other people in the world, and the return on that investment is negative. We have higher rates of obesity, heart disease, diabetes, shorter life expectancy and higher infant mortality rates than even some "third-world" countries.[14]

Before I go any further, let me be abundantly clear about one thing—I am not against all forms of medicine and medical practice. Remember, my

Gramps was a high-profile member of the medical community. Tracy is a registered nurse. She has worked in surgery for most of the time I have known her. Certain drugs and surgeries have their place and always will.

I have a good friend who is a surgeon at a trauma center in a major city. One day we were talking about the problems in the American medical system and he said, "America has the greatest trauma centers in the world. If you are involved in a car wreck or shot or stabbed or are involved in any kind of trauma, there is no better place in the world to be. But, if you want to stay well, stay away. If you get sick we're nearly as likely to kill you as heal you."

My friend was right. Do you know what disease is the third most fatal in the United States? It's Iatrogenic Disease.[15] Ever heard of it? I hadn't until recently. Iatrogenic Disease is defined as a disease that is caused by medical treatment, and it claims the lives of approximately 250,000 Americans a year.[16] [17]

Again, don't misunderstand me. I am not pointing the finger at individuals. This is about a system that is broken. Doctors and nurses can only work with the tools and information they are given. Too often, their hands are tied. When they speak up about problems they see, they are often bullied into silence for fear of losing their jobs. When you begin to dig into what is behind the medical industry, you run into large multinational companies whose practices make those of the food industry pale by comparison.

Perhaps the biggest problem is that the medical community is controlled by the pharmaceutical industry. Medical technology and pharmaceuticals are rapidly changing. What doctors learn in medical school is usually obsolete before they even graduate. Once they get into practice they tend to rely on salespeople. These specialized sales people tend to be young, attractive, charismatic and of the opposite sex. I had a friend in Memphis who was a sales manager for a pharmaceutical company and he confessed that was exactly who he was taught to recruit.

Again, I am not blaming these individuals. They are only doing what they have been taught. The doctors are grossly overworked. They are under a lot of stress and pressure. They don't have time to do the research. So when these companies send in their reps and wine and dine them and offer financial incentives, it's just easier to go with the flow. They trust what they are told.

Like the food industry, the drug companies also have slick advertisements. We see a television commercial that urges us to talk to our doctor about XYZ drug, so we do. When you walk into your doctor's office, you feel like you're supposed to walk out with a prescription. You know, the one you saw on TV with that really happy person with the perfect life and the serene music. But there's a problem. Taking those prescriptions hospitalizes approximately 1.9 million people a year and will kill approximately 128,000 people.[18] That's not people who died from an overdose or took the wrong drug or made a mistake. That's more than 100,000 deaths a year from known side effects.

You read that correctly. Millions of people are hospitalized and more than a hundred thousand die every year because they took drugs exactly as prescribed. And you thought all of those side effects listed at the end of the commercial were just to cover the industry's rear end. When I see those commercials, I usually think that I'd rather have the condition than the side effects.

I'll give you just one example, and you can probably extrapolate from there. Have you seen those commercials for heartburn and acid reflux medications? I'm sure you've seen the one for "the purple pill." In these commercials, you often see someone looking forlornly at some favorite food they can't eat, such as pizza or burgers or whatever. Then they say something like, "Thanks to XYZ drug, I can still eat my favorite foods."

It's not that simple.

Those drugs are called proton-pump inhibitors and they reduce the production of acid by blocking the enzyme in the wall of the stomach that produces acid. That's a problem. You need that acid to break your food down into smaller molecules. Normally the pH of the acids in your stomach is around 1.75 - 2.0. That's up there with battery acid. Within a couple of weeks on being on a proton-pump inhibitor, the pH goes up to around 5. That's the pH of coffee. What would you rather have breaking your food down — battery acid or coffee?

This means your food is not being broken down very well which leads to other problems. For one thing, you stop being able to absorb nutrients as well. One listed side effect is bone density issues. That's because you're not getting enough magnesium, so you're at higher risk of bone fractures. You are at higher risk of kidney disease. It also increases your risk of diseases from infection. You also have a 10.5 fold increase in food allergies and sensitivities.

I'll just toss this little nugget out and you can do what you want with it. When I was in my first-year Greek class in seminary I ran across the word *pharmakeia* in Galatians 5:20, which is translated "sorcery." It is defined in Thayer's Greek-English Dictionary as *"the use or the administering of drugs; poisoning; sorcery, magical arts, often found in connection with idolatry and fostered by it."*[19] Strong's Greek Dictionary defines it as:

"medication ("pharmacy"), i.e. (by extension) magic (literally or figuratively): — sorcery, witchcraft."[20]

As you may have already guessed, *pharmakeia* (sorcery) is a form of the Greek root from which the English words pharmacy and pharmaceutical are derived. According to noted New Testament Greek scholar Kenneth Wuest, the "word speaks in general of the use of drugs, whether helpfully by a physician, or harmfully by someone whose purpose it is to inflict injury, hence, in the sense of poisoning."[21] Another renowned Greek scholar W.E. Vine said *pharmakeia* "primarily signified 'the use of medicine, drugs, spells'; then, 'poisoning'; then, 'sorcery,'"[22] Vine went on to say, "In 'sorcery,' the use of drugs, whether simple or potent, was generally accompanied by incantations and appeals to occult powers, with the provision of various charms, amulets, etc., professedly designed to keep the applicant or patient from the attention and power of demons, but actually to impress the applicant with the mysterious resources and powers of the sorcerer."[23]

The book of Revelation reveals that sorcery will take place in the end times on a large scale and will be used to enslave the nations. Speaking of the fall of Babylon the Great, John wrote, "your merchants were the great ones of the earth, and all nations were deceived by your sorcery" (Revelation 18:23 ESV). There also appears to be a connection here between *pharmakeia* and extremely powerful merchants. Keathley commented, "The word "sorcery" is singular and looks at a whole program of sorcery or deception, a world conspiracy by the merchants or super rich magnates in control of the commercial system of Babylon, the multinational corporation heads. . . . This states in effect that the Babylonian system will use whatever method it can to poison the minds of men and to deceive them."[24]

The range of definitions for *pharmakeia* allows for both good and bad uses. Are there medications that are good and useful? Certainly. For example, Ezekiel mentions using the leaves of fruit trees for healing (Ezekiel 47:12). Of course, that's a natural plant-derived remedy. Still, I believe there are good and legitimate uses of drugs and medications.

That being said, pharmaceuticals can also harm and even kill—they do so quite often. And what about the big multinational pharmaceutical companies? Are they seeking your best interests or their own?

Like I said, do what you want with that information. Pray about it. Ask God to speak to your heart. I'll leave it alone for now—that's a whole other book. I will say this though, if you are trusting in a "magic potion" to relieve you of the symptoms of your life choices instead of following God's plan to give you health and heal you, I would say that falls into the category of "works of the flesh." Wouldn't you?

ENEMIES WITHIN

> But he turned and said to Peter, "Get behind me, Satan! You are a hindrance to me. For you are not setting your mind on the things of God, but on the things of man."
>   —JESUS (Matthew 16:23 ESV)

We are now awake to the fact that we have an enemy who throws every weapon he has against us to destroy us and rob us of the life we were meant to live in Christ. Peter showed us that our enemy is a roaring lion. Paul revealed that our struggle is against spiritual forces. We know that these forces are behind a world system of institutions that want to deceive and manipulate us.

It is good to know these things. Ignorance is *not* bliss, and what you don't know *can* kill you. But there is another enemy we need to identify. That enemy is ourselves. The greatest enemies of God's people have always been internal and not external.

That should be obvious. Our external enemy is defeated. "He [God] disarmed the rulers and authorities and put them to open shame, by triumphing over them in him [Christ]" (Colossians 2:15 ESV). Our enemy has no power and no authority over us—except what we give him.

And there it is.

Turn back with me to the first book of the Bible and re-read the story of The Fall. Satan twisted God's words to deceive Adam and Eve, which led to an open rebellion against God. While Adam blamed Eve, and Eve blamed the serpent, their excuses didn't fly.

Now flip back to the end of your Bible and read the letters to the churches in Revelation 2–3. Jesus never condones false teachings outside the church, but His primary concern for these churches is that some of them were holding to immoral practices (Revelation 2:14 ESV), and heretical teachings (2:15).

To the church at Thyatira He says, "I have this against you, that you tolerate that woman Jezebel, who calls herself a prophetess and is teaching and seducing my servants to practice sexual immorality and to eat food sacrificed to idols" (Revelation 2:20 ESV). God is merciful and gave her time to repent, but she refused. So, He said He would throw her onto a sickbed and throw those who follow her into great tribulation (2:21-22).

We—the church in America—are too much like the Church at Laodicea. Jesus has a message for us:

> I know your deeds, that you are neither cold nor hot; I wish that you were cold or hot. So because you are lukewarm, and neither hot nor cold, I will spit you out of My mouth. Because you say, 'I am rich, and have become wealthy, and have need of nothing,' and you do not know that you are wretched and miserable and poor and blind and naked, I advise you to buy from Me gold refined by fire so that you may become rich, and white garments so that you may clothe yourself, and that the shame of your nakedness will not be revealed; and eye salve to anoint your eyes so that you may see. Those whom I love, I reprove and discipline; therefore be zealous and repent. Behold, I stand at the door and knock; if anyone hears My voice and opens the door, I will come in to him and will dine with him, and he with Me. (Revelation 3:15–20 NASB)

When Jesus said, "Behold, I stand at the door and knock," He was speaking to the church. Not the world. Not the lost. He was pointing out that the greatest threat to the church does not come from the outside, but from the inside. Our greatest threat is our own unwillingness to hear and obey the Word of God—and whether we will succumb to the teachings of our enemies.

As long as we're looking in the mirror, let's have a look at the first chapter of Romans. That's where Paul took His readers—including us—on a proverbial trip behind the wood shed. He started out in verse 18, "The wrath of God is being revealed from heaven against all the godlessness and wickedness of people, who suppress the truth by their wickedness," (NIV). Then, for the rest of the chapter, he let loose a scorching condemnation against sin and humanity's suppression of truth. But he saved the most crushing blow for last, and he aimed right at the heart of the church—those who should know better, but don't. Are you ready for this? "Though they know God's righteous decree that those who practice such things deserve to die, they not only do them but give approval to those who practice them" (Romans 1:32 ESV).

The greatest enemy of God's people comes from within. If we take ourselves out, who will go and share the love of Christ to a lost and dying world. And who would want our lives anyway? We only have something to offer the world if they can see a difference in us. They have to see something they want.

The world needs us at our best and that means we start with the person we see in the mirror. It's where God always starts—with His people.

FRIENDLY FIRE

Do you remember what I said in the introduction about Dana warning me that the greatest opposition to this ministry would come from within the church? He was right. But that's not really surprising is it? The worst blows in life tend to come from those who are the closest to us and should love us the most—our family and friends. Often, their opposition is born out of misunderstanding. Remember the story of David and Goliath? David was only a youth. He was untrained for war. His father had him out tending the sheep.

But his father sent him to the frontlines to take food to his older brothers. That's when he heard the taunts of the Philistine champion, Goliath. And that got David fired up. Even though he wasn't a trained warrior yet, he knew God would deliver Goliath into his hands with only a sling and a few stones.

But David's oldest brother misunderstood the situation and accused David of being an arrogant, irresponsible, wicked little brat. Sounds like family, doesn't it?

Even Jesus dealt with it. "So his brothers said to him, 'Leave here and go to Judea, that your disciples also may see the works you are doing. For no one works in secret if he seeks to be known openly. If you do these things, show yourself to the world.' For not even his brothers believed in him" (John 7:3–5 ESV).

Dana's experience was that people opposed him because of the style of music he played. The song "Don't Stop the Music" was a response to the anti-"Christian rock" movement spearheaded by evangelist Jimmy Swaggart. As believers, we don't have to agree on everything. Yes, there are essentials to the Christian faith—salvation by faith alone through grace alone in Christ alone, for example. But there is also a saying often attributed to Saint Augustine, "In Essentials Unity, In Non-Essentials Liberty, In All Things Charity."

Just as the Christian rock movement and contemporary worship movement have seen opposition from within the church, the faith-based fitness movement has seen its share of opposition. A few years ago, I created a video for YouTube called "Faith and Fitness." I received an email one day from a pastor in West Virginia named Steve Willis. A friend of his had seen my video and asked him if he knew me because we were saying some of the same things. So Pastor Willis reached out. He had been on Jamie Oliver's *Food Revolution* show and had written a book called *Winning the Food Fight*. He had been interviewed on national TV shows on both Christian and secular networks. We ended up talking on the phone for a couple of hours.

At one point, I told Steve about my conversation with Dana and asked if he had experienced that kind of opposition himself. "Absolutely," he said. "Talking about the sin of gluttony and how we are killing ourselves with food in the church is not very popular. Too often the church doesn't want to hear it."

It's a topic that hits a little too close to home. Perhaps it's because it's a sin we can't very well hide—it bulges out right there in front of us. I know because mine did. It's a sensitive subject, but sometimes we need a little tough love.

I've told pastor friends that if they think it's tough to preach a message on tithing, they ought to try teaching one on food addiction. I've been called Pharisee, I've been accused of being legalistic. I've had people cover their plates when I walk up so I won't see what they're eating. I've heard things like, "Now don't judge me for eating this ____ (fill in the blank)."

For starters, I'm not judging. It's not my place. I may feel bad for someone because I know the consequences they will face, but that just prompts me to love and pray for them more. What I've often wanted to say, but never have—at least not out loud—is, "It's not me you should be worried about. You should be more concerned about the One whose temple you are destroying with your choices."

I know—it's kind of harsh. That's why I haven't said it to anyone. I'm saying it now, though. Oh, and just so you understand that we're on a level playing field, I say that to myself too.

We had great success running Fit Clubs in churches. We would get together once a week, sometimes twice, and work out together. Usually, it was as simple as putting in a workout DVD and everyone doing that together. Sometimes I would lead a live workout. Sometimes, we would run challenge groups with weekly weigh-ins and celebrations for the victories we accomplished. We celebrated those who lost weight, worked out so many days in a row, or made healthy choices. We shared recipes, and we shared struggles. We prayed for each other, and we invited people in from the community. It was awesome!!

What's more, God moved. He broke down strongholds in people's lives. We shared the gospel, and people who had not been in church, sometimes in years, came back to God and began walking with Him. You see, when you meet a physical need and love someone through their pain, you earn the right to share your faith. They want to know.

Still I would occasionally hear of people who thought what we were doing was absolutely horrible. How dare we do something as "fleshly" as work out in church. How dare we teach people that God cares about their health and fitness. We were accused of damaging people's self-image and teaching people to think they had to be thin to please God. We were reminded that God loves us just like we are, and that people get enough negative messages from the world.

Of course, God loves us. But that doesn't mean He wants us to stay where we are. Let's change the subject. Instead of obesity and food addiction, let's use that logic on alcoholism. You see where it breaks down? Yes, God loves us. Does He love the alcoholic? Absolutely. Sin doesn't change that. But He still doesn't like the sin. So, should we keep silent and leave the alcoholic to their addiction so we don't offend them? Nope.

That would be the most unloving thing we could do. The loving thing is to help them overcome it, to help them heal and find freedom. Isn't that what God has called us to do?

As God's people, we are far too easily pleased. We settle for far less than God's best and pretend we are being pious. Phooey! We must get out of this rut we have dug for ourselves. We must claim our rightful place as sons and daughters of God! As A.W. Tozer has said,

> Everything Jesus Christ did for us we can have in this age. Victorious living, joyous living, holy living, fruitful living, wondrous, ravishing knowledge of the Triune God—all of this is ours. Power we never knew before, undreamed of answers to prayer—this is ours. "See, I have given you this land. Go in and take possession of [it]." The Lord gave it to you in a covenant. Go take it - it's yours."[25]

CHAPTER 3

FIGHT FOR YOUR LIFE

What we do in life echoes in eternity.[1]
   —MAXIMUS (*Gladiator*)

Sometimes you need to get hit in the head to realize that you're in a fight.[2]
   —MICHAEL JORDAN

We don't need another diet book. We aren't lacking for books telling us what we should or shouldn't eat or how important exercise can be. It's not that we don't have at least a general idea of *what* to do. What we lack is a deep understanding of *why* it matters.

Maybe it's because we haven't been hit in the head yet.

That's what it took for me. It took being diagnosed with pre-diabetes and impending heart disease for me to wake up and fight back. I pray you wake up sooner than I did, or at least that you wake up before it's too late. Because it's not really diabetes and heart disease and cancer you are risking, is it? It's what those diseases will cost you.

Health is like wealth. By itself, wealth is nothing. Money is not an ends; it is a means to an end. Nobody hoards money because of what it is, but because of what it means to them. Scrooge wasn't miserable because he hoarded money. He hoarded money because he was miserable. Scrooge had a broken, twisted heart.

Health is the same way. Having a lean, fit body is nice, but it is not the goal. It's a side effect. The goal is to be fully alive for the glory of God. I imagine you already understand that, by definition, you can't be fully alive if you are not at optimal health—much less if you are suffering from the side effects of an undisciplined life.

The Apostle Paul said, "I discipline my body and keep it under control, lest after preaching to others I myself should be disqualified" (1 Corinthians 9:27 ESV). Why did he do that? What was the point of disciplining his body? There is a principle in psychology that says all human behavior is motivated by two things: either seeking pleasure or avoiding pain. It's the carrot or the stick. Paul shows us both.

> "I do all things for the sake of the gospel, so that I may become a fellow partaker of it. Do you not know that those who run in a race all run, but only one receives the prize? Run in such a way that you may win. Everyone who competes in the games exercises self-control in all things. They then do it to receive a perishable wreath, but we an imperishable. Therefore I run in such a way, as not without aim; I box in such a way, as not beating the air; but I discipline my body and make it my slave, so that, after I have preached to others, I myself will not be disqualified" (1 Corinthians 9:23–27 NASB).

The first thing Paul told us was that he did *all things* for the sake of the Gospel. He glorified God with every aspect of his life: "So, whether you eat or drink, or whatever you do, do all to the glory of God" (1 Corinthians 10:31, ESV). Even when he was in prison awaiting death, he proclaimed, "For to me to live is Christ, and to die is gain. If I am to live in the flesh, that means fruitful labor for me" (Philippians 1:21-22 ESV). Paul was looking forward to Heaven. He couldn't wait to get there. He had endured hardships and persecution and torture. Yet, he longed to live so that He could accomplish more for Christ.

From there, Paul made his point by using the ancient Olympics as an example. I love watching the Olympics with my family. We watched the 2016 Summer Olympics together and marveled at the skill, grace, and talent of such world-class athletes. That year, our favorites were swimmer Michael Phelps and gymnast Simone Biles. Their skill and dedication were awe-inspiring. They are shining examples of what the human body can accomplish.

Our bodies are amazing machines that God has given us. We are truly "fearfully and wonderfully made" (Psalm 139:14, ESV). Of course, Olympic athletes are on a different level than probably 99.9 percent of people. They are set apart. But, then again, so are we.

We are set apart to serve God. Like Olympians, we can accomplish so many great things when we discipline ourselves daily over a period of years. As Paul said, we need to exercise "self-control in all things."

I think that's why Paul used athletes as an example. I think he wanted us to take something familiar and transpose it to a higher key. You may have noticed athletes and athleticism are often used to convey deeper spiritual truths. That's because the same fundamentals and disciplines apply to every area of our lives—even 2,000 years later.

For example, one thing I noticed in my own life is that when I became more disciplined with my body, I also became more disciplined in other areas of my life. That was certainly true of my spiritual life. I believe that is the overarching principle Paul wanted us to catch. When we see elite athletes in action, it should arouse within us an overwhelming desire to fight the good fight and run the race of life with nothing less than the passion and purpose of an Olympic athlete.

In his commentary on the New Testament, Albert Barnes points out that the commitment of most Christians pales when compared to the dedication of Olympians:

> How much their conduct puts to shame the conduct of many professing Christians and Christian ministers. They set such a value on a civic wreath of pine or laurel, that they were willing to deny themselves, and practise [sic] the most rigid abstinence. They knew that indulgence in WINE [sic] and in luxurious living unfitted them for the struggle and for victory; they knew that it enfeebled their powers, and weakened their frame; and, like men intent on an object dear to them, they abstained wholly from these things, and embraced the principles of total abstinence. Yet how many professed Christians, and Christian ministers, though striving for the crown that fadeth not away, indulge in wine, and in the filthy, offensive, and disgusting use of tobacco; and in luxurious living, and in habits of indolence and sloth! How many there are that WILL [sic] not give up these habits, though they know that they are enfeebling, injurious, offensive, and destructive to religious comfort and usefulness. Can a man be truly in earnest in his professed religion; can he be a sincere Christian, who is not willing to abandon anything and everything that will tend to impair the rigour of his mind, and weaken his body, and make him a stumbling-block to others?[3]

Why do we struggle with self-control when athletes who don't follow God do whatever is necessary to accomplish their goals? We have a far more powerful motivation than any athlete. They do it for what is temporary; we do it for what is eternal. The manner in which we run and fight has eternal consequences. Remember, eternal does not mean future. It means unending. So, our life choices produce consequences for better or worse, and those consequences start now. How we live demonstrates whom and what we are placing our faith in, what our true values are, and what is closest and dearest to our hearts.

Life is the proving ground—not of what we can do in our own strength, but for what we can do through His strength. I love what John Piper said:

> Life is not a field for demonstrating the force of our will to make good choices. It's a field for showing how the beauty of Christ takes us captive and constrains us to choose and run for his glory. The race of life has eternal consequences not because we are saved by works, but because Christ has saved us from dead works to serve the living and true God with Olympic passion (Hebrews 9:14).[4]

Ironically, Hollywood gets it right sometimes—as the character Maximus said in the Ridley Scott epic *Gladiator*, "What we do in life echoes in eternity."[5] We are not earning our place in eternity. We are proving that we already have it. As the brother of Jesus said, "I will show you my faith by my works" (James 2:18, ESV). It is not enough to think right or believe right. Our faith needs to transform how we live. It needs to affect how we run, how we fight. Honestly, our salvation doesn't depend on the way we discipline our bodies, but our discipline is evidence we are saved—because faith without works is dead (James 2:18-28).

Paul's use of Olympic athletes as an example was genius. They prepare their entire lives for one moment. They get one shot at a gold medal. One. So when they run, they run to win—and there is only one winner. They run hard. They give absolutely everything they have. Everything. There are no do-overs. This is it.

That's the example Paul used. Therefore, he said "Run in such a way that you may win."

We've lost a bit of that in our culture. My oldest son, Reese, is a baseball player. He's only 12, but he talks about wanting to play in high school and college. That means he starts preparing now.

A couple of local coaches who work with elite players have been hosting winter workouts for anybody who wants to come. It has been so good for Reese. He's getting to hang out with and practice with boys who are older and more experienced, including a couple of young men who are playing in college. He's working with coaches who love the game and love pushing young men to become their best. When the boys run sprints, these coaches yell at the boys to give it everything they've got. You see, you will play the way you practice.

What Reese is just beginning to learn is how much work it takes to be an elite athlete. It's a tough lesson. Until now, he has played little league ball where everybody on every team gets a trophy. We don't want to hurt anyone's feelings; we think it builds their self-esteem.

It doesn't.

Speaking on the issues that Millennials are facing in the workplace, author Simon Sinek has said, "Some kids got participation medals. They got a medal for coming in last. Right? The science we know is pretty clear, which is it devalues the medal and the reward for those who actually work hard. And it actually makes the person who comes in last feel embarrassed, because they know they didn't deserve it, so it actually makes them feel worse."[6]

The reality of life is you get nothing for coming in last. We have an entire generation that has no idea what it's like to push themselves to their absolute limits. They've never had to, and it's getting them into trouble.

Paul told us to give nothing less than our best. Because we run to bring honor and glory to Christ, we should run with passion, purpose, and intensity. Not lazy or listless or lethargic or mindless. Run to win—which is why we exercise control in all things (9:25).

Now, I know what you're thinking: *He's just trying to step on toes. All things? Seriously? Come on, don't we get to slack off somewhere?* To be honest, you can slack off if you want—but only at the risk of being disqualified.

Paul concluded, "So I do not run aimlessly; I do not box as one beating the air. But I discipline my body and keep it under control, lest after preaching to others I myself should be disqualified" (1 Corinthians 9:26–27 ESV). So much for our comfortable, lukewarm lives. Paul says that exercising self-control is like running, not without aim, but with our eyes on the course. It's like boxing, but not shadow boxing or throwing punches at the air. He meant boxing that connects with a target. In this case, his target was his body. One version says, "I'm landing punches on my own body and subduing it like a slave" (CEB).

He didn't do this because the body is essentially bad like the dualists believed. On the contrary, the body is good. God created it. And as we'll see in a little bit, He will raise it again one day to live forever. No, Paul disciplined his body because our sin nature tempts us to give in to appetites that run contrary to God's will for our lives. Paul would never allow himself to be enslaved to the tyranny of momentary pleasures. His eye was always on the prize.

Paul understood that the appetites and desires of the flesh are not easily subdued. That's why he used such severe language. He also knew that if we discipline our bodies and bring them under control, the reward will be far greater than anything we "give up." And here's the real kicker—you will learn (as I did) that you won't even want the things you once thought you couldn't live without. You'll discover that there is far greater reward in doing things God's way—not just in the hereafter, but right here and right now: "Truly I tell you," Jesus said to them, "no one who has left home or wife or brothers or sisters or parents or children for the sake of the kingdom of God will fail to receive many times as much *in this age*, and in the age to come eternal life." (Luke 18:29-30 NIV *emphasis mine*)

There is nothing you can sacrifice that you will not receive back many times over. Jesus once told His followers, "Give, and it will be given to you. They will pour into your lap a good measure—pressed down, shaken together, and running over. For by your standard of measure it will be measured to you in return" (Luke 6:38 NASB). If you want to receive all that God has for you, you have to give Him everything. Your spirit. Your soul. Your body.

PROTECT THIS HOUSE

Glorify God in your body.
— THE APOSTLE PAUL (1 Corinthians 6:20 ESV)

Take care of your body. It's the only place you have to live.[7]
— JIM ROHN

Physical fitness is not only one of the most important keys to a healthy body, it is the basis of dynamic and creative intellectual activity.[8]
— JOHN F. KENNEDY

Now may the God of peace himself sanctify you completely, and may your whole spirit and soul and body be kept blameless at the coming of our Lord Jesus Christ.
— THE APOSTLE PAUL (1 Thessalonians 5:23 ESV)

The first time Sarah came over to our house, she said that she wanted to know whether or not God really cared about her body.

"Show me," she said. "I have to see it."

Sarah needed more than proof-texts. She wasn't interested in anyone else's "interpretation" of what God says. What Sarah wanted and needed was to be walked through the Bible so she could see and know and understand for herself what God says about our bodies.

Sarah fully believed that God had sent her to us. She knew there was something He wanted her to learn from us, and she was beginning to sense that she was being called to a level of life that required her to get her body firing on all cylinders. But she was a skeptic.

Actually, "seeker" is probably a better word. She had her doubts, but she was open to learning. Sometimes, skeptics already have their minds made up, so there's no point in confusing them with the facts. And that's irritating, to put it mildly. But a seeker admits there are things they don't know, so they're seeking that knowledge. I love seekers.

Sarah has a hunger for God and for truth, and she has no problem submitting to the will of God once she knows it. But first she needed to be convinced in her own mind that her health and fitness mattered to God.

That's perfect. It's not my place to convince her, or you, of anything. Honestly, it's beyond my ability and not worth the time either of us would need to invest. You see, if I have to convince you, you'll never own it; therefore, your habits won't change—at least not long term. It's much better for you to see and be convinced for yourself.

Luke commended the people of Berea because, while they eagerly received Paul's message, they also "examined the Scriptures every day to see if what Paul said was true" (Acts 17:11 NIV). So please, don't take my word for it. See for yourself.

So where should we start? How about where God started—at the beginning. Literally. The very first verse of the Bible begins the account of creation: "In the beginning, God created the heavens and the earth" (Genesis 1:1 ESV). The pinnacle of creation is the creation of humanity—male and female—because we were created in God's image: "Then God said, "Let Us make man in Our image, according to Our likeness . . . God created man in His own image, in the image of God He created him; male and female He created them" (Genesis 1:26-27 NASB). Men and women both bear the image of God, each in their own unique way. But at our core, we are triune in nature, just as He is. God is triune in nature—the Trinity. Three-in-one, Father, Son, and Holy Spirit. Man is also triune—body, soul and spirit.

Notice the language. "God said, 'Let *Us* make man in *Our* image, according to *Our* likeness'" (1:27). The phrasing here is intentional. God is speaking to Himself—to the Trinity: God the Father, God the Son, and God the Holy Spirit. They are coequal, coeternal, three distinct persons, yet one God. And all three are present here. In the creation account, the Spirit of God is moving, and God the Father is speaking, while Jesus is creating. How do we know this? Because Paul and John both say so. Speaking of Jesus, Paul said, "For by him all things were created, in heaven and on earth, visible and invisible, whether thrones or dominions or rulers or authorities—all things were created through him and for him"

(Colossians 1:16 ESV). That's pretty awesome, but what John said in the opening of his Gospel, is simply poetic: "In the beginning was the Word, and the Word was with God, and the Word was God. He was in the beginning with God. All things were made through him, and without him was not any thing made that was made" (John 1:1-3 ESV). Did you catch that. Jesus is the Word. He was *in the beginning* with God—the exact opening words of Genesis—"In the beginning, God—Jesus—The Word created ..." All things! Everything! Man, that's exciting!

That should fill you with wonder and awe! In fact, let's just sit in that for a moment. It was Jesus at creation who formed Adam from the dust of the ground (Genesis 2:7) and gave him a physical body. I imagine a master sculptor at work. Lovingly and carefully, he set about molding and shaping Adam's body. I think He took His time. I picture Him singing as He worked. I think He delighted in the masterpiece He was creating. And I believe He did the exact same thing when he knit you together in your mother's womb.

How does that thought make you feel?

But God wasn't done yet. Next, God breathed the breath of life into Adam's nostrils. Sort of like divine CPR, I suppose. There was no breath in Adam, so God gave him His breath. What is God's breath? It is the Spirit. The Hebrew word for spirit is *ruach*, which means "wind, breath, air, spirit." We don't know for sure that this is a reference to the Holy Spirit, but it seems evident that this set Adam apart from the rest of creation. There is no record that God breathed into any other creatures. It is at this point that Adam became a "living being"—he woke up and saw the face of his Creator. Adam was now eternal and triune—created in the image of God.

God later created woman from Adam's side. Both were created in God's image—both in their own unique and special way. Both had a body, soul, and spirit. They would also pass this image on to their offspring—to us.

We are not spiritual beings trapped in an earthly body, as some would have you believe. Our body is as much a part of who we are as our soul and spirit. As Paul wrapped up his first letter to the Thessalonian church he prayed for them: "Now may the God of peace make you holy in every way, and may your whole spirit and soul and body be kept blameless until our Lord Jesus Christ comes again" (1 Thessalonians 5:23 NLT). Paul was referring to the totality of human nature, which includes the body. His desire for the church was for every aspect of their being to be kept blameless. He also had absolute confidence that God, who is faithful, would do it. And He will—at the coming of our Lord Jesus Christ.

You see, when Christ returns, He will resurrect our bodies. We don't get a new one. We get the same one, only restored to perfection. I'm hoping that means I get a full head of hair. But the point is, we retain our physical body in Paradise. God fully restores us to what we were intended to be. We aren't just spirits floating around in the afterlife. We are physical.

Jesus was called the "firstborn from the dead" (Colossians 1:18; Revelation 1:5) and He had a physical body after His resurrection. This was the same physical body complete with the scars from the nails and spear—only perfected. But until that day, God has entrusted the care of our bodies and soul and spirit to us.

It is very much like the relationship between God and a farmer. A farmer trusts God for a harvest. He is completely reliant on God to provide the soil and sun and rain and the miracle of life, but he must do his part. He must till the soil and plant the seeds and care for the plants. You would think a farmer who blamed God for a lack of a harvest for a crop he never planted or cared for was a fool. Why would you think it is any different with our bodies?

In His Word, God has given us everything we need to know about the proper care of our bodies. We will dig into the details of that later, I promise.

Being an image-bearer of the Most High God is both highly motivating and incredibly serious. It is not something to be taken lightly. You probably already realize that, but maybe you're still not quite convinced that your body bears the image of God. Think of it this way: Do you know why murder is such a big deal? Because it destroys what was created in the image of God. In fact, God takes it so seriously He prescribes the death penalty for murder for that very reason. "Whoever sheds the blood of man, by man shall his blood be shed, for God made man in his own image" (Genesis 9:6 ESV). Murder does not harm the soul or the spirit—only the body. Therefore, the punishment relates to a crime against the image of God in the body.

Here's something else to ponder: If you kill another human being without just cause, it's called murder. If you kill yourself, it's called suicide. What do you call it if you kill yourself—if you cut your life short—through an unhealthy lifestyle? You know you should eat better, but you don't. You know you should get more exercise, but you don't. "So whoever knows the right thing to do and fails to do it, for him it is sin" (James 4:17 ESV).

If you're like me, that hits pretty close to home.

God is our "Abba Father"(Romans 8:15; Galatians 4:6). It is this name for God that gives us perhaps the most profound insight into how He relates to us. *Abba* is an Aramaic word that is most closely translated as

"Daddy." It was the familiar term young children used for their father. He lovingly created us—created our bodies. Like any good father, He wants only the best for us. I can understand that because that's how I feel about my children—and I only played a minor role in their creation compared to God's role. He's the One who knits us together in our mother's womb (Psalm 139:13). We are truly fearfully and wonderfully made in His very image (Psalm 139:14).

That's why He wants to make us holy in every way: spirit and soul and body. Because He loves us, He wants us to be complete. Like the Trinity, our three parts are equal and interconnected. To neglect any one of them leaves us incomplete. It would be like neglecting one leg of a 3-legged table. Without all three legs in balance, the table won't stand and can't be used for its intended purpose.

We are the same. We cannot pick and choose areas of our life to give to God. It all belongs to Him. We are pretty good about encouraging each other to take care of soul and spirit, but we tend to neglect our body. The problem is, doing that negatively affects the other two areas. But when we learn to discipline our bodies—which really is a spiritual discipline—we find that we become disciplined in other areas. When God controls every area of our lives, we are complete and can honor Him completely.

That brings me to the next point—we were created to bring God glory. In Isaiah, God refers to His sons and daughters as, "Everyone who is called by My name, and whom I have created for My glory, whom I have formed, even whom I have made" (Isaiah 43:7 NASB). Whenever you begin to doubt your worth, consider what God says about you here. He created you for His glory.

He didn't say He wanted us to *increase* His glory, or somehow make Him more glorious. It doesn't work that way. He is *God.* He is, was and ever will be perfect, complete, and holy. And He created us to *display* His glory—to make His glory *known* and *praised.*

Our bodies are a marvel—no, a mystery—of engineering. For all of our modern science we still don't know exactly how it all works. And we certainly can't create anything even remotely close to it ourselves.

AN ACCEPTABLE VICE?

Sadly, our lack of concern for this wonderful and marvelous body—this gift from God—has become the norm. In some cases, we might even view anyone who takes care of their body as a little crazy. Meanwhile, we make excuses for our own over-indulgence in food and lack of exercise. We say things like, "We don't live under the law, but under grace." Of course, we do live under grace. We find God's forgiveness through grace (Ephesians 2:8-9). But when it comes to how we are living, well, it's really just an excuse. It's not even original! Paul dealt with the same argument in the church at Corinth.

> All things are lawful for me, but not all things are profitable. All things are lawful for me, but I will not be mastered by anything. Food is for the stomach and the stomach is for food, but God will do away with both of them. Yet the body is not for immorality, but for the Lord, and the Lord is for the body. . . . Do you not know that your body is a temple of the Holy Spirit who is in you, whom you have from God, and that you are not your own? For you have been bought with a price: therefore glorify God in your body. (1 Corinthians 6:12-13,19-20 NASB)

To be completely fair, this is not an easy passage to interpret. We live in a different time and culture than the first-century Corinthians, so we have to work through those differences to understand the nuances as they did. The big picture, though, is quite clear. It boils down to who has authority over our bodies. Paul started out by correcting the Corinthians misapplication and abuse of Christian liberty. He then drove his point home with absolute certainty: Our bodies belong to Christ, purchased by His blood and accountable to His lordship. Paul then pulled everything together with the command: "glorify God in your body."

As Oswald Chambers said in *My Utmost for His Highest*:

> I am accountable to God for the way I control my body under His authority. Paul said he did not "set aside the grace of God"— make it ineffective (Galatians 2:21). . . .What I must decide is whether or not I will agree with my Lord and Master that my body will indeed be His temple. Once I agree, all the rules, regulations, and requirements of the law concerning the body are summed up for me in this revealed truth-my body is "the temple of the Holy Spirit."[9]

Every activity related to our bodies must be understood in light of these truths. For the Corinthians, food was part of the problem. It seems the more things change, the more they stay the same. Centuries ago, Solomon put it this way, "What has been is what will be, and what has been done is what will be done, and there is nothing new under the sun" (Ecclesiastes 1:9 ESV). Our struggles are nothing new.

So, Paul needed to correct the Corinthians' views about freedom. While we are free in Christ, that freedom is ultimately for God's glory—not a license to pursue pleasure wherever it leads us. As he said in verse 12, a lot of things were lawful, but they weren't all profitable.

Commentators and translations generally agree that, "all things are lawful for me" was a popular and convenient slogan among Corinthian Christians.[10] They used their "freedom" from the law as a license to do whatever they wanted. The Pillar Commentary on 1 Corinthians says, "It is clear that some Corinthians were asserting their freedom to do certain things that Paul objected to—here, involving prostitution; in chapter 10, eating food explicitly identified as having been offered to idols."[11] But I love how Paul revealed how their "logic" was actually self-defeating—not just once, but twice. Paul never disagreed that "all things are lawful." He knew it was true to a certain extent. As a child of God, all of our sins—past, present and future—have been washed away and covered by the blood of Christ. God has separated them from us as far as "the east is from the west" (Psalm 103:12 ESV). Nothing can separate us from the love of God (Romans 8:38-39).

It's also true that God created us to enjoy His creation, including food. But that freedom is not absolute. God sets boundaries both to protect us and to increase our delight and pleasure.

So, instead of arguing the point, Paul simply added an obvious and pertinent truth—"not all things are profitable." Some things simply aren't in our best interests—or the interest of others. These days, we'd call that a "Duh!" moment. It seems so obvious: Just because you *can* do a thing doesn't mean that you *should*. Yet, all of us can think of times when we just didn't think it through.

Paul's second exception was a little stronger: "All things are lawful for me, but I will not be mastered by anything." He flipped the script and revealed another paradox of freedom. As Elton Trueblood said, "We have not advanced very far in our spiritual lives if we have not encountered the basic paradox of freedom . . . that we are most free when we are bound. ... Discipline is the price of freedom."[12] Boom! Paul slammed the door on this presumptuous argument by revealing that their alleged freedom actually led them right back into bondage. Far from being the master of their bodies, they were mastered by desires that undermined and opposed their higher purpose and calling.

God's freedom isn't just freedom *from* something. It's also the freedom *for* something. In our default condition, we are slaves to sin (2 Peter 2:19). But through Christ, we can choose to be slaves of righteousness. We have to choose our master wisely. As Bob Dylan poignantly observed in the song, *Gotta Serve Somebody*, we will either serve the devil or serve the Lord, but ultimately we're going to serve somebody.[13]

Paul's first task was to help the Corinthians (and us) understand that while we are free to choose our actions, we are not free to choose the consequences of those actions. Every decision has a consequence, good or bad. We must constantly ask ourselves if something is allowable. But we also have to ask if it's profitable and whether it's mastering us.

From there, Paul shifted gears and got very practical: "Food is for the stomach and the stomach is for food, but God will do away with both of them" (6:13). As it turned out, he was right on track, since the Corinthians used the slogan "all things are lawful" to justify all kinds of appetites. In fact, the ancient world regularly linked an appetite for food with sexual appetites. According to Roy Ciampa and Brian Rosner, "There is considerable evidence in pagan, Jewish, and Christian writings that feasting and sexual immorality went together."[14] Ancient texts indicate that sexual pleasure was often the expected after-dinner entertainment of a banquet, including engaging in the services of prostitutes.[15] While that wouldn't go over at your next church potluck, it was apparently fairly normal in first-century Corinth.

The Corinthians misunderstanding regarding food and sex was rooted in their misguided belief that the spirit is sacred and the physical body is corrupt and inconsequential—what we defined earlier as "dualism." We still see this misconception pop up in our churches today from time to time—especially with food. Like the Corinthians, we often believe that a physical act, such as eating, has no moral significance. We can eat whatever we like without consequence.

Ironically, most of us are appalled when this idea is applied to sexual immorality—sleep with whomever you want whenever you want. But we use the same argument to justify abusing our bodies with food and sedentary living. The truth is we, like the Corinthians, want to do what we want to do, and we'll justify it by putting a spiritual spin on it.

Paul corrected the Corinthian belief that the body is just moving toward ultimate destruction by reminding them that the body belongs to the Lord. And just like God raised Jesus' body from the dead, He will also raise our body. Our bodies aren't destined for destruction, they're scheduled for glorification! They aren't disposable; they're recyclable.

Is that really how you view God's amazing gift of your body? That's exactly what Paul challenged the believers in Corinth to understand.

The heart of the disagreement between Paul and the Corinthians concerned the value of our physical existence in the present age—whether or not our body matters. Paul sought to correct their misunderstanding and thereby change their behavior. The body is not insignificant or temporal. On the contrary, it is incredibly valuable and will one day be raised to new life. And since it has eternal value, how we behave now is important.

But Paul was just warming up.

After making the case that our freedom in Christ is not a license to sin, that our bodies are eternal, and that what we do with them matters, Paul built on the foundation he had already laid by launching into an imaginary debate with the Corinthians.

In verse 15, Paul asked, "Do you not know that your bodies are members of Christ?" In his own tongue-in-cheek way, Paul was saying that if they had really known it, they would have behaved differently. Understanding that their bodies were joined with Christ would have prevented the Corinthians from going so far astray. This "do you not know" is the sixth of 10 times in 1 Corinthians that Paul used the phrase to remind them of something that he clearly feels they should have known (3:16; 5:6; 6:2, 3, 9, 15, 16, 19; 9:13, 24). It's the fourth time in chapter 6 alone—with two more coming up. In other words, this is no longer a polite reminder. Paul was clearly peeved and moved from simply asking questions to forcefully rebuking his readers. Their (and our) ignorance is inexcusable.

Paul then rhetorically asked, "Shall I then take away the members of Christ and make them members of a prostitute?" The answer is obvious, right? Paul certainly thinks so, because he answered emphatically, "May it never be!" No! Absolutely not! His whole argument was based on his belief that our spirit, mind, and body are connected—that we are created in God's image and, like Him, are one being with three distinct parts. What we do with one part affects the whole, and you can never be fully alive if you are not whole.

More than that, Paul's words remind us that at the moment of salvation, we became united with Christ—including our bodies. He is with us wherever we go and whatever we do.

Now, before we can go any farther, I need to address a common objection I get with these verses. Obviously, Paul is specifically addressing sexual immorality here, so many think that these verses cannot be used to promote physical fitness or to police what we eat. I've even had a pastor tell me that the verses only apply to what you eat if you are having sex with your food. Seriously? Would it surprise you to know that he was obese?

The truth is, we will go to any lengths to justify our behaviors, and the Corinthians were a perfect example of that. The overarching point of these verses is summed up in verse 20, "therefore glorify God in your body." The specific examples he provides are food and sex. And, for our purposes, we can't forget that Paul obliterated the idea that what we eat is irrelevant (v. 13).

Paul used the issue of immorality along with food because the Corinthians were dealing with both temptations. Prostitution was completely acceptable in Greek and Roman cultures; and, as strange as it seems to us, some of the Corinthian Christians may have been regularly engaging with prostitutes. But the fact that it was commonplace didn't make it right.

Likewise, it's common for Christians in America today to approach food in ways that weaken and destroy the body resulting in gluttony, rampant obesity, and disease. I'm pretty sure Paul would be just as incredulous at our lack of understanding of how our habits are a sin against our own bodies and against Christ.

The real issue is the incompatibility of light and darkness—the battle between what belongs to God and what opposes God. Paul's argument was based on that incompatibility. In 1 Corinthians 10:14–22 and 2 Corinthians 6:14–7:1, Paul used the same logic to demonstrate that whatever is opposed to God is, by nature, demonic. Whether it's going to prostitutes, eating food sacrificed to idols, or being unequally yoked with unbelievers, the Corinthians were renouncing the lordship of Christ over their bodies, denying their resurrection life to come, and acting in ways that harmed Christ's body.

Paul's heart, and therefore God's heart, was broken. He wanted to impress upon us a high view of our bodies and all the behaviors that concern it. When he wrote to the Philippians, he said, "For many, of whom I have often told you and now tell you even with tears, walk as enemies of the cross of Christ. Their end is destruction, their god is their belly, and they glory in their shame, with minds set on earthly things" (Philippians 3:18–19 ESV). You can almost see him writing with tears in his eyes and with a heart broken over those who allow their appetites to control them—individuals walking as enemies of the cross of Christ.

The last thing any believer would ever want to be said of them is that they are enemies of the cross of Christ! We need to seek God's forgiveness. We need to ask Him to open our eyes and to help us to walk with Him, not against Him.

Paul's attack against their behavior prompted him to fire off another "do you not know" and his reasoning of why sex with a prostitute is absolutely unthinkable, because it joins the believer's body with that which is offered to demons. Many people today, as in Paul's day, believe in the notion of casual sex. There is no such thing as casual sex. The assumption here is that every sexual act fuses the two partners together into one flesh.

Which leads Paul to his emphatic command "flee immorality!" He will later plead with us to "flee idolatry" (1 Corinthians 10:14-31) in relation to eating pagan foods. The two commands are linked. As one commentator pointed out, "The two, idolatry and sexual immorality, are intertwined in Paul's mind." and "As a union with a prostitute is unthinkable for a Christian, so becoming a partner at a table with demons is equally unthinkable."[16]

Paul wraps up with a stirring crescendo—the all-encompassing argument for the high value of the body in verses 19-20: You just can't get around the truth in these verses. God Himself takes up residence within every believer. And, since our bodies are the temples of the Holy Spirit, they are set apart to display the awesome glory of God.

Every phrase here is cruise missile aimed at the heart of the Corinthians' defenses. *Your body is a temple of the Holy Spirit who is in you.* In every religion, temples are regarded as sacred and holy. It's a glorious privilege that we are a temple of God, but it also carries the most serious of obligations to keep that temple pure. Imagine how upset you would be if someone backed a manure truck up into your church and dumped the whole load into the sanctuary.

First and foremost, abusing our appetites—whether physical or sexual—is wrong because our bodies do not belong to us. They are marked for God by the Holy Spirit and reserved for His purposes.

Paul added that we *have been bought with a price.* The imagery here comes from the ancient slave market, another concept familiar to the Corinthians.[17] This is not a picture of a slave being bought by God and being set free, but being transferred by sale from one owner to another. Formerly we were slaves to sin, now we are slaves of God (Romans 6:16-23; 7:6).

Therefore, we're commanded to glorify God in our bodies. To engage in any behavior that damages our bodies, not only defiles the temple of the Holy Spirit, but also rejects the life God has given us. The decisive question is, Who really owns your body?

Which takes us back to the question posed to us by Oswald Chambers—will we agree with our Lord and Master that our body will indeed be His temple?

Where do you stand?

CHAPTER 4

THE HEART OF WORSHIP

I appeal to you therefore, brothers, by the mercies of God, to present
your bodies as a living sacrifice, holy and acceptable to God, which
is your spiritual worship. Do not be conformed to this world, but be
transformed by the renewal of your mind, that by testing you may
discern what is the will of God, what is good and acceptable and
perfect.
    —THE APOSTLE PAUL (Romans 12:1–2 ESV)

We only learn to behave ourselves in the presence of God.[1]
    —C.S. LEWIS

He who would accomplish little must sacrifice little; he who would
achieve much must sacrifice much; he who would attain highly
must sacrifice greatly.[2]
    —JAMES ALLEN

Does the Lord delight in burnt offerings and sacrifices
    as much as in obeying the Lord?
 To obey is better than sacrifice,
    and to heed is better than the fat of rams.
       —THE PROPHET SAMUEL (1 Samuel 15:22 NIV)

Worship is a way of gladly reflecting back to God the radiance of
His worth.[3]
    —JOHN PIPER

More than three-quarters of a century ago, on June 8, 1941, as his
nation was engulfed in a desperate war against Adolph Hitler and the
Nazis, and enduring the near continual bombardment of the Battle of
Britain, C.S. Lewis, the renowned British author and scholar, climbed the

steps of the University Church of St. Mary the Virgin in Oxford and delivered one of the most profound sermons of the twentieth century. He titled it *The Weight of Glory*, from 2 Corinthians 4:17, "For our light affliction, which is but for a moment, is working for us a far more exceeding and eternal weight of glory" (NKJV). In the face of a very real military enemy and the horrors of war, Lewis began with a rather surprising premise—that sacrifice, as demonstrated through unselfishness, is not the greatest virtue. This introduction has become one of his most famous passages. Lewis began by stating if you asked twenty good men what the highest virtue was that they would reply unselfishness, but if you had asked the same question of any of the great Christians of old they would have replied love. Love, of course, is the correct answer. It was the answer Jesus gave (Matthew 22:36-40). Lewis then points out that somehow a positive idea got replaced by a negative one and how that carries with it the suggestion that what we give up is more important than any good it might do. Self-denial, he says, is not an end to itself. In fact, every time we are told to deny ourselves in the New Testament, it contains an appeal to our desire. Desire is not a bad thing, it is good, and Lewis submitted that any notion that desire is bad "has crept in from Kant and the Stoics and has no part of the Christian faith." Lewis then laid down one of the most profound recriminations of the modern church that echoes the words of Jesus to the church at Laodicea.

> Indeed, if we consider the unblushing promises of reward and the staggering nature of the rewards promised in the Gospels, it would seem that Our Lord finds our desires, not too strong, but too weak. We are half-hearted creatures, fooling about with drink and sex and ambition when infinite joy is offered us, like an ignorant child who wants to go on making mud pies in a slum because he cannot imagine what is meant by the offer of a holiday at the sea. We are far too easily pleased.[4]

It seems contradictory to talk about worship and pursuing our own desires in the same breath, until you understand *true* worship. Worship is not about sacrifice, at least not in the way we usually think about it. Worship is not as much about what we give up as about what we gain. It is a response of love—we love Him because He first loved us (1 John 4:19).

That's why the prophet Samuel said, "to obey is better than sacrifice" (1 Samuel 15:22). God desires obedience that is motivated by love, not forced or coerced. You are probably familiar with the phrase, "God loves a cheerful giver," but do you know the context of that verse? It was Paul who said, "So let each one give as he purposes in his heart, not grudgingly or of necessity; for God loves a cheerful giver" (2 Corinthians 9:7 NKJV). It was an encouragement to obey with a heart moved by love and gratitude, not duty.

As a father, I understand this. It brings great joy to my heart when my children obey happily and willingly—because they love me and understand that my heart is always seeking their good. One of my greatest joys as a father comes when my children spontaneously hug me or crawl up in my lap to tell me how much they love me.

In a sense, that is the heart of worship. God smiles when we act out of pure, unbridled love for Him. As Piper said, "The real duty of worship is not the outward duty to say or do the liturgy, it is the inward duty, the command: 'Delight yourself in the LORD!" (Psalm 37:4). 'Be glad in the LORD and rejoice!" (Psalm 32:11). The reason this is the real duty of worship is that it honors God, while the empty performance of ritual does not."[5]

Are you beginning to get a picture of what God desires in His relationship with us? The example of a parent and child is a nice one, but not quite adequate. We've probably been asleep too long and become overly concerned with being "proper." As a result, we've lost the passion, enthusiasm, and intimacy we were designed to enjoy. We might need to be shocked to wake up to what God is trying to tell us. That's just how God rolls.

To give us a glimpse of how our union with Christ is supposed to work, Paul pointed to the relationship between a husband and wife. Writing to the church at Ephesus, he quoted Genesis and delivered a shocker out of what seems like left field: "For this reason a man shall leave his father and mother and shall be joined to his wife, and the two shall become one flesh. This mystery is great; but I am speaking with reference to Christ and the church" (Ephesians 5:31–32 NASB). How's that for scandalous? How's that for passionate? Paul just used the explicitly sexual imagery of a husband and wife becoming one flesh as a picture of the relationship between Christ and His bride, the Church. That's me and you.

Think about it, though, there is no other union on earth that so completely stirs our passions and emotions as the consummation of the love between a husband and wife. There is no deeper and intense connection. As John Eldredge said in *The Journey of Desire*:

> People don't jump off bridges because they lost a grandparent. If their friend makes another friend, they don't shoot them both. No one has ruined home and career for a rendezvous at the library. Troy didn't go down in flames because somebody lost a pet. The

passion that spousal love evokes is instinctive, irrational, intense, and, dare I say, immortal. As the Song says, Love is as strong as death, its jealousy unyielding as the grave. It burns like a blazing fire, like a mighty flame. Many waters cannot quench love; rivers cannot wash it away (Song 8: 6– 7).[6]

The Bible is the greatest romance ever written. It is the story of the all-powerful, all-knowing God who created humanity in His image and for intimacy with Himself. Our sexuality is a living metaphor for why we were created. God's design for marriage is that the "two shall become one flesh." We are designed to crave the level of intimacy that interweaves two into one.

Is this difficult to imagine that level of intimacy with God? Too often, we relegate God to some distant corner or shelf as something to be respected and honored and revered, instead of letting our hearts come alive with excitement and anticipation of worship—kind of like it did on our wedding night. Our hearts need to burst with love and a passion to worship our Creator and Savior—not just for an hour on Sundays, but throughout the week.

Lewis was right, "The Lord finds our desires, not too strong, but too weak. . . We are far too easily pleased."

If you're struggling to see how this relates to our bodies, let me pull back on the reins a little and give you a "PG" example. Tracy and I were married on November 19, 1999. I was accidentally wise to select that date because it's pretty easy to remember—11/19/99 (or 111999).

But I digress.

Suppose I plan a perfect anniversary. I book a getaway for us at a beautiful resort, set her up for the day at the spa to be completely pampered, take her to a romantic dinner, followed by a walk on the beach, talking, laughing, celebrating our lives together. We finally get back to our room, and she blushes as she tells me how perfect the day was and how loved she feels.

Then, I respond with, "Don't mention it. I was just doing my duty as your husband."

How do you think the rest of the night will go?

Exactly. So, why do you imagine God, who loved you so much He gave His Only Son to ransom you, would take any pleasure in you doing anything for Him because you feel obligated? It's like a slap in the face.

So, how are we supposed to apply all of Paul's talk about presenting our bodies as sacrifices and our spiritual act of worship? Obviously, Paul didn't mean that our bodies are a sacrifice for sin. Christ already paid that debt with His body. Instead, he meant that we should gladly demonstrate our love for Christ in how we use our bodies.

And notice, Paul was making an "appeal," not issuing a commandment. He was making an urgent invitation—an exhortation.

And this appeal is based on a "therefore." As I learned in a college Bible study, anytime you see a "therefore" in Scripture, you should stop and ask yourself, "What's that therefore there for?" In other words, take a look at what came before the "therefore" so you'll have the proper context. In this case, that would be the first eleven chapters of Romans, which describe our sin, Jesus' sacrifice, and the decision we're all called to make. But Paul just nicely summed it all up for us in the phrase, "by the mercies of God."

In light of our depravity and inability to save ourselves, Christ, in His mercy, willingly sacrificed His body on our behalf. So, with that love and mercy as a backdrop, is it really so much for Christ to ask us to offer our bodies to Him? Piper is a little more blunt: "The point here is not to present to God your bodies and not your mind or heart or spirit. He is going to say very clearly in verse two: 'Be transformed in the renewal of your mind.' The point is to stress that your body counts. *You belong to God soul and body, or you don't belong to him at all.* Your body matters" (*emphasis mine*).[7]

Now, let's go back and think about that word *sacrifice* a little more—and give it a definition we can work with. One dictionary defines it as, "an act of giving up something valued for the sake of something else regarded as more important or worthy."[8] But that idea of sacrifice isn't really a sacrifice, is it? If I tell you I will give you $100 bill in exchange for your $1 bill, that's a pretty good deal—at least for you. You'd be crazy not to "sacrifice" your dollar for 100 times more! But what God is offering holds infinitely greater value.

Paul urged us to offer something we value—our bodies—in exchange for something of far greater value—the opportunity to worship Him and enjoy Him forever. Taking the time and money to invest in a wonderful, romantic anniversary with my wife is not mere duty. It is a joy and pleasure. It would be just a small token of how much I love her and of her great worth to me. I gladly offer her my life.

How much more should we offer our lives to the One who rescued us from sin and death? Who gave us both our physical life and our spiritual life. Oh, and I'm pretty sure that Tracy would freely offer her body to me because of her love for me and in response to my love for her—not because it was her "duty."

When we offer our bodies as a living sacrifice, we honor the One who gave us life. It also acknowledges a transfer of ownership. Remember Paul's exhortation in 1 Corinthians 6:19-20? Jesus paid a price for us, so we are called to glorify God in response. Paul said something of a transfer also occurs in marriage: "The wife does not have authority over her own body, but the husband does; and likewise also the husband does not have authority over his own body, but the wife does" (1 Corinthians 7:4 NASB).

Now, before you start getting upset about the imagery of slavery and submission—and start looking for that verse about freedom in Christ—keep this in mind: Your supposed freedom can lead you right back into a different kind of slavery. That's why Paul reminded us, "For you were called to freedom, brothers. Only do not use your freedom as an opportunity for the flesh, but through love serve one another" (Galatians 5:13 ESV). And again, "Once, you offered the parts of your body to be used as slaves to impurity and to lawless behavior that leads to still more lawless behavior. Now, you should present the parts of your body as slaves to righteousness, which makes your lives holy" (Romans 6:19 CEB).

As a child of God, I have the privilege of offering my body as a living sacrifice to gladly show Jesus how much I love Him—to give Him all the glory, honor and praise. Every day, I get to choose to be a part of God's plan and purposes here on earth, to be His hands and feet, and to have His power working through my body. As Paul said, "for me to live is Christ" (Philippians 1:21 NIV).

That kind of sacrifice begins with our health and fitness. It's not that God wants us to be fitness models or athletes—though He can and does use both. It's because He wants us to be tools He can use to accomplish His purpose.

Do you remember the 2004 Indian Ocean earthquake and tsunami that devastated more than a dozen countries, including Indonesia, Sri Lanka, India and Thailand? Somewhere between 230,000 - 280,000 people died in that tragedy. The images and videos of the destruction were overwhelming.

We were attending Germantown Baptist Church at the time, and our pastor, Sam Shaw, was a former missionary. Our church sent people and resources to Indonesia to lend whatever aid we could and to share the love of Christ. I vividly remember Pastor Shaw telling the congregation that he believed every Christian should have a passport. That way, when an event like that occurred, we could immediately go if God called us.

I absolutely agree 100 percent! And allow me to add this: Every Christian should be as physically healthy and strong as possible for the same reason. Please hear what I am saying. I know some things are out of your control. But control what you *can* control. As much as it depends on you, be as healthy as you can be. God is not as concerned with your ability as your availability, so be available.

For example, you can control what you eat. You can control the amount of physical activity you get (based on your ability). You can control your mindset. You can control what and who influences you.

Sound like drudgery? Are you thinking about what you will have to give up? Is there a voice deep down inside saying you can't do it? That's the enemy lying to you.

Remember, we are at war. Paul knew that. That's why he wrote, "Do not be conformed to this world, but be transformed by the renewal of your mind" (Romans 12:2 ESV). We've got to learn how to recognize the voice of our enemy and rebuke him with the Word of God: "I can do all things through him who strengthens me" (Philippians 4:13 ESV). Transform negative thoughts into positive truth. That's what C.S. Lewis was talking about—we've substituted negatives for positives and been too easily satisfied with the results! Instead of telling yourself, "I *have* to eat healthier," or "I *have* to get more exercise," change it to "I *get* to—I have the opportunity to worship God through my choices."

DO YOU WANT TO BE HEALED?

Have you noticed that Jesus always knows the exact right question to ask? It's because He knows our hearts. He knows our truest and deepest desires, even if we forget. Yes, His questions are disruptive, but they're meant to be. One of my favorite examples is found in the fifth chapter of John's Gospel.

> Some time later, Jesus went up to Jerusalem for one of the Jewish festivals. Now there is in Jerusalem near the Sheep Gate a pool, which in Aramaic is called Bethesda and which is surrounded by five covered colonnades. Here a great number of disabled people used to lie—the blind, the lame, the paralyzed. One who was there had been an invalid for thirty-eight years. When Jesus saw him lying there and learned that he had been in this condition for a long time, he asked him, "Do you want to get well?" "Sir," the invalid replied, "I have no one to help me into the pool when the water is stirred. While I am trying to get in, someone else goes down ahead of me." Then Jesus said to him, "Get up! Pick up your mat and walk." At once the man was cured; he picked up his mat and walked. (John 5:1-9 NIV)

The Pool of Bethesda had become a dumping ground of sorts for broken people. There had been a rumor going around for who knows how long that an angel would come down from time to time and stir up the water. When that happened, the first person to get in would be healed.

It's probably just a legend, mind you. The earliest manuscripts don't contain this detail. It was apparently added in later to give some context to the man's conversation with Jesus. Still, the story was popular enough that it attracted a crowd of hopeful people—each one thinking that day would be *their* day for a miracle. Among the crowd was a man who has been sick for 38 years. We don't know exactly what his illness was, only that it apparently left him unable to walk. So there he was, lying in a sea of humanity . . . waiting.

Enter Jesus. Once He saw the man and learned that he had been lying there for so long, the Lord asked him a simple question: "Do you want to get well?" Older translations read, "Will you be made whole?"

Hold the phone. What did Jesus say? Did He ask a man who had been sick for 38 years, was lying next to the pool of Bethesda, and hoping to be the lucky first person into the water if he wanted to get well? You would think the answer was obvious.

Imagine if you were in the man's shoes and Jesus had asked you the same question. I know how I'd be tempted to respond: *Do I want to be healed? What kind of stupid question is that? Of course, I want to be healed! I've been lying here for years! What do you think? Are you completely insensitive?*

But Jesus wasn't being insensitive. He loves us more deeply than we can ever begin to imagine. And it wasn't a dumb question because Jesus never asks dumb questions. Instead, it was a question with purpose! Jesus asked because He knew the man had a deeper issue that needed to be addressed. Perhaps He was addressing a fundamental truth of human nature: illness, disease and other problems don't automatically result in a sincere desire for healing or improvement.

Perhaps Jesus was really asking something deeper: *Do you really want things to change? Are you ready to quit making excuses? Are you ready to take on the responsibilities of an improved life?* Many people say that they want better health or a better quality of life, but they resist the change. They want to keep doing the same things that got them where they are—and then they marvel that their lives don't improve. I've heard that doing the same thing over and over and expecting different results is one definition of insanity. So, why do we do it? Why do we act so crazy? Because in order to change, we first have to admit that we are responsible. We also have to do things that can be uncomfortable—or even painful. So, it feels easier to just remain as we are.

Of course, it could have been that the man was suffering from what motivational speaker Zig Ziglar used to call "P.L.O.M. disease" (Poor Little Ol' Me). Not everybody who asks for help is actually looking for a solution. Believe it or not, a lot of people don't want to get well. They make a show of wanting things to be better; but when push comes to shove, their true desires are betrayed by their action—or rather their inaction. Sadly, they have grown comfortable with their afflictions. All they really want is attention and sympathy. If you foul up the deal and solve their problem, they can't complain about it anymore.

Whatever was going on, the man's answer revealed that Jesus had hit the nail right on the head! You can tell because the man didn't answer the question. He began to make excuses instead. He didn't have any help. Someone always beat him into the water. Rather than accept responsibility, he gave explanations: "It's not my fault, and here's why . . ."

On the surface, his excuses might sound reasonable—until you consider who else Jesus had healed. There was the blind beggar in Mark 10:46-52 who made an absolute scene as Jesus walked by, shouting at the top of his lungs and begging Jesus to have mercy on him—despite the crowd telling him to hush. And there was the paralyzed man in Luke 5:18-25. His friends carried him to Jesus; and, when they couldn't get into the house, they tore a hole in the roof and lowered him down. Or what about that woman in Luke 8:43-48—the one with the blood condition who pushed her way through the crowd just to touch the hem of Jesus' robe as He walked by?

I could go on, but I think you see the point.

I don't know about you; but if I *really* believed those waters would have healed me, I would have figured out a way to get into that pool when the waters were stirred. I would have camped out right on the water's edge and rolled in as soon as I saw the first ripple. I would have found someone to help me, like the paralytic whose friends tore up the roof. I would have at the very least yelled and screamed at Jesus as he walked by like the man in Mark 6. I would have done *something*.

But there is no record that this man did any of those things. He just lay there in his misery. Wishing. Blaming.

To be fully alive as God intends, we must be honest with Him and with ourselves. We have to recognize that we are broken. We have to see and acknowledge our pain. We must accept responsibility for what is within our control. We must dare to hope for a miracle.

And did I mention that Bethesda means "House of Mercy?"

Jesus, God Incarnate, offered just that—mercy and grace in the form of a command. He interrupted the man's pity party and told him to take action: "Get up, take up your bed, and walk." As soon as he did what he was told, the man was healed. He picked up his bed and walked.

God offers us life. He interrupts the narrative the enemy is speaking into our lives. He dismisses our excuses and replaces them with words of life.

Like every other story in the Bible, this is God's story. The primary focus of this passage is declaring the amazing grace, mercy and power of Jesus Christ. This miracle is all about Christ—from start to finish. He was the One who first noticed the paralyzed man, not the other way around. And it was Jesus who spoke first. He supplied not only the will and the power to be healed, but He also commanded the man to take up his bed and walk.

That's my Jesus!

But there's another lesson for us to take from this miracle—one that demonstrates a very human response to change. We tend to resist change. After all, it's so much easier to blame people or circumstances than to take responsibility and do what is necessary to change. What does this passage say to us? Stop being a victim of your circumstances!

Don't get me wrong. I am not criticizing the paralyzed man. I know—and the Lord knows—that I'm just like him in so many areas of my life. So are you. But the good news is that we don't have to be.

You see, the very same power that healed this man and raised Christ from the dead is available to us. Earlier, I mentioned Philippians 4:13: "I can do all things through him who strengthens me." But to release that strength, you have to take action. To have a productive harvest, you have to prepare the ground, plant the seeds, and care for the plants. Change occurs the moment you decide what you really want and commit to do whatever it takes to achieve it.

THE JOY OF STEWARDSHIP

If you could do better, should you?[9]
   —JIM ROHN

God, grant me the serenity to accept the things I cannot change,
Courage to change the things I can,
And wisdom to know the difference.[10]
   —THE SERENITY PRAYER (REINHOLD NIEBUHR)

An elderly man trudges slowly, purposefully, along a path overlooking the coastline. His family follows a slight distance behind. His posture and face let us know that his soul carries a heavy burden. His eyes fill with tears as the wave of emotions continues to build. The American and French flags flapping in the breeze give us a clue to where he is: The Normandy American Cemetery.

The man is obviously a veteran—someone who knows too well the sacrifices and tragedies of war. He turns and begins walking through the rows of crosses that mark the graves of American heroes. He is here on a mission. He is here to pay his respects.

Finally, he finds the headstone he's looking for and falls to his knees weeping. The memories come flooding through his mind, taking him back to June 6, 1944.

You may remember this as the opening scene of Steven Spielberg's epic movie, *Saving Private Ryan*. Two hours and forty minutes later we learn that the man is Private James Ryan. The name on the cross: Capt. John H. Miller. This is the man he came to pay his respects to, the man he came to thank for his life. You see, Captain Miller gave his life to save Private Ryan, and the last words he said to him were: "James . . . earn this. Earn it."

As Ryan kneels in front of the grave he begins to speak. He tells Captain Miller that every day of his life he has thought about those final words. He says he has tried to live his life the best he could. He hopes it has been enough. Captain Miller's words have haunted Private Ryan for decades. They motivated him to live every day with purpose, to always do his best. And yet, still he is haunted by doubt.

When his wife walks up, he turns and says to her, "Tell me I've lived a good life. Tell me I'm a good man." She cradles his head in her hand and says, "You are." It is a poignant ending to a powerful drama—and a stark reminder to make every moment count.

Although I disagree theologically with the premise that we could ever *earn* the sacrifice God made on our behalf, I do believe that we should all ask ourselves if we are living a life that *honors* His sacrifice. Which brings us to a question Jim Rohn has asked: "If you could do better, should you?" As a follower of Christ, the answer should be obvious.

According to Jesus, the first and greatest commandment is, "you shall love the Lord your God with all your heart and with all your soul and with all your mind and with all your strength" (Mark 12:30 ESV). Jesus' sacrifice demands that we surrender everything to Him—every aspect of our lives and of our being. When Jesus called His disciples, He called them to leave everything and follow Him.

Excellence, then, is not an option for those who claim to be followers of Christ. It's an imperative. Regarding the difficulty of the Christian life, C.S. Lewis commented:

> The Christian way is different: harder, and easier. Christ says "Give me All. I don't want so much of your time and so much of your money and so much of your work: I want You. I have not come to torment your natural self, but to kill it. No half-measures are any good. I don't want to cut off a branch here and a branch there, I want to have the whole tree down. I don't want to drill the tooth, or crown it, or stop it, but to have it out. Hand over the whole natural self, all the desires which you think innocent as well as the ones you think wicked—the whole outfit. I will give you a new self instead. In fact, I will give you Myself: my own will shall become yours.[11]

Did you catch that part about no half-measures being any good? That's exactly what the resurrected Jesus told the church of Laodicea in Revelation 3:14-16. This was a church that had grown comfortable and complacent. Essentially, He reminded them that there is no place for half-heartedness in the kingdom of God. To paraphrase the Savior's words: *You're either all in or you are out. Your mediocrity and unwillingness to surrender everything and live life to your fullest potential makes Me want to throw up.*

In his book, *The Pursuit of Holiness,* Jerry Bridges draws an interesting parallel between spiritual and physical warfare. He asks:

> Can you imagine a soldier going into battle with the aim of 'not getting hit very much?' The very suggestion is ridiculous. His aim is not to get hit at all! Yet, if we have not made a commitment to holiness without exception, we are like a soldier going into battle with the aim of not getting hit very much. We can be sure if that is our aim, we will be hit—not with bullets, but with temptation over and over again.[12]

In our daily pursuit of holiness our goal should be to honor God with everything we do, even the little things. "So, whether you eat or drink, or whatever you do, *do all to the glory of God*" (1 Corinthians 10:31 ESV, *emphasis mine*). Things that may seem insignificant in the here and now can have far-reaching—even eternal—consequences.

In Luke 9:23 Jesus said, "If anyone would come after me, let him deny himself and take up his cross daily and follow me. For whoever would save his life will lose it, but whoever loses his life for my sake will save it" (ESV).

Did you catch that? The only way to save your life is to give it up. The glorious truth is that when we fully surrender our lives to Christ, God will use us in ways we never dreamed were possible. We do not have to be famous or particularly gifted. We simply have to be willing and faithful. I've heard it said that God does not need your ability, just your availability.

And when God called you to follow Him, He did not leave you alone. He provides all of the strength and resources you'll ever need to accomplish the tasks he has set before you (Phil 1:6; 4:9,13). God calls us to make the most of what we have been given. We should faithfully and joyfully do all that He asks.

That's what it means to be a wise manager, a steward, of all that He has entrusted to us. As Paul said, "This is how one should regard us, as servants of Christ and stewards of the mysteries of God. Moreover, it is required of stewards that they be found faithful" (1 Corinthians 4:1–2 ESV). "Steward" is not a term we use a lot in our culture. The closest word we have is probably "manager." But it refers to those who have been given a trust—a responsibility—to faithfully care for a master's possessions placed in their care.

Peter put it this way, "As each has received a gift, use it to serve one another, as good stewards of God's varied grace" (1 Peter 4:10 ESV). We are called to be faithful and wise managers of the gifts and resources God has given us. That includes our bodies.

When we consider what it means to be faithful stewards of all God has entrusted to us, we must first start with ourselves—our bodies. We have to surrender our bodies to the Lord before we can fully give Him our time, our talents, our money, and our relationships. When we maintain optimal health and fitness, we are in a better position to effectively use all the other gifts He has given us. After all, giving our time or money doesn't mean much unless we have already given ourselves. More than anything, actually, the Lord wants us. He wants our love, our hearts, our very lives. Our service, our hard work, is no substitute for all we are.

Which takes us back to our original question, slightly modified: "If you could do better with your health and fitness, should you?" Again, the obvious answer is, "Yes!" You cannot live life to the fullest if you are not in good health, and that means being physically fit inside and out.

Dr. Stan May, one of my seminary professors, used to say, "There are only two days that matter—this day and that day. And on *that* day you will give an account for *this* one." One of the things we'll give an account of on that day is how we managed our bodies, God's temple.

Now, I know what you're thinking: *That's all fine and good, but you don't know my circumstances.* Well, you're right. I don't. But I also believe it doesn't matter because we are only responsible for what we've been given.

Between His resurrection and His Ascension, Jesus took a walk with Peter along the beach (John 21:15-23). As he and Jesus spoke, Peter looked back and saw John walking behind them. So, he asked, "Lord, what about this man?" Basically, Jesus told Peter to stop worrying about John and to focus on keeping his own feet on the right path.

That's the way stewardship works. It's personal. It's individual. And nobody else is responsible for what you have been given—and you're not responsible for what they have either.

We see this in the Parable of the Talents (Matthew 25:14-30). A master entrusted different amounts to each servant, each according to his own ability. When he returned from the trip, what each man had been given was the standard by which he was judged—and blessed.

SERVING OUR LORD

"For it will be like a man going on a journey, who called his servants and entrusted to them his property. To one he gave five talents, to another two, to another one, to each according to his ability. Then he went away. He who had received the five talents went at once and traded with them, and he made five talents more. So also he who had the two talents made two talents more. But he who had received the one talent went and dug in the ground and hid his master's money. Now after a long time the master of those servants came and settled accounts with them. And he who had received the five talents came forward, bringing five talents more, saying, 'Master, you delivered to me five talents; here I have made five talents more.' His master said to him, 'Well done, good and faithful servant. You have been faithful over a little; I will set you over much. Enter into the joy of your master.' And he also who had the two talents came forward, saying, 'Master, you delivered to me two talents; here I have made two talents more.' His master said to him, 'Well done, good and faithful servant. You have been faithful over a little; I will set you over much. Enter into the joy of your master.' He also who had received the one talent came forward, saying, 'Master, I knew you to be a hard man, reaping where you did not sow, and gathering where you scattered no seed, so I was afraid, and I went and hid your talent in the ground. Here you have what is yours.' But his master answered him, 'You wicked and slothful servant! You knew that I reap where I have not sown and gather where I scattered no seed?

Then you ought to have invested my money with the bankers, and at my coming I should have received what was my own with interest. So take the talent from him and give it to him who has the ten talents. For to everyone who has will more be given, and he will have an abundance. But from the one who has not, even what he has will be taken away. And cast the worthless servant into the outer darkness. In that place there will be weeping and gnashing of teeth.'" (Matthew 25:14–30 ESV)

Let's break this down a little bit. Jesus set the scene by telling us that a man, Luke called him a nobleman (Luke 19:12), entrusted his estate to his servants while he was away on a long journey. To one he gave five talents, to another two, and to the third he gave one. Each, Jesus said, received an amount "according to his ability."

How much is a talent worth you ask? That's a good question. A talent was a first-century weight measurement for gold or silver. In the Roman Empire, a talent was approximately 33 kilograms. According to goldprice.org, the price of gold today, March 25, 2017 is $40,024 per kilogram. At that price, one talent would be worth approximately $1.32 million. Now, although the original audience would have understood the word "talent" in financial terms, this parable is the origin of the sense of the word "talent" meaning "gift or skill" as used in English and other languages.[13] Pretty cool, huh?

And did you catch that part about each being given a different amount according to his ability? God gives us exactly what we can handle—no more, no less. And, as we discussed earlier, that is all we are responsible for.

This is also true of our health, isn't it? Have you ever met someone who, no matter what they eat or how much, never seems to gain a pound? Doesn't that frustrate you? There are some people who seem to be born with a natural fitness and athletic ability while others struggle. Some people are more prone to illness while others never get sick. No matter what we have been given, we are responsible for it, no more and no less. The important thing to remember is that we are judged based on what we did with what we were entrusted—not how much we ended up with. The great thing about this is that, unlike people, God is never impressed with numbers. He is impressed with faithfulness.

All of us are called to live up to our fullest potential, by God's strength, with His wisdom, and for His kingdom. Everything that we have comes from God; therefore, our stewardship includes everything: our time, talents, gifts, personality, experience, attitudes, material resources, energies, and, yes, our bodies.

What does this mean for us when it comes to being good stewards of our bodies? It means God does not need you to be a supermodel or super-athlete unless that is His calling on your life. There is no need to compare yourself to others or to compete with them. Your only concern is to be faithful with what God has given you to the best of your ability.

For the sake of time, I'll skip to the end of the story—that's the important part anyway. The man returned from his journey and called the servants together. He was eager to hear their reports, and, to be fair, the first two guys did pretty well. They had invested their master's money and had doubled their investment. As a result, they were both rewarded with more. (vv. 21, 23).

But the third servant didn't do so well. He returned the one talent he had been given to his master. Nothing lost—but nothing gained either.

At least he could account for all of it, right? Wrong. His one talent was taken from him and given to the guy who already had 10. And as if that wasn't insult enough, he was thrown out in the darkness where "there will be weeping and gnashing of teeth" (25:30). Whoa! What? All he did was hide his master's money. He didn't lose it. He was just playing it safe—the path of least risk and resistance. But his excuses revealed his heart. He was afraid of his master. He didn't trust the master's heart. Clearly, he didn't really know his master. He was exposed as wicked and lazy—so he lost everything.

I have often wondered why the one given the least turned out to be the bad guy in this story. Jesus was not implying that those who are entrusted with less will automatically be unfaithful. But He was saying that even if you have only been entrusted with a *little*, you are responsible for it. No matter how much God gives you, you're responsible to create a return on His investment.

There are some people whom God has given privilege after privilege, yet they let it all go to waste. Others receive very little, but they use it well. Perhaps Jesus used the man with the one talent to represent the wicked servant to show that the master's anger wasn't related to how much money was lost. He was angry because the servant wasted his opportunity.

The question you have to ask yourself is, *What kind of servant am I?* It has been said that our potential is God's gift to us, while what we do with it is our gift to Him. Zig Ziglar once put it this way, "You are the only person on earth who can use your ability." Are you investing in your health, so that you can live longer, live better and be more useful to God? Or are you literally digging your own grave by neglecting your body?

The issue here is not about what was lost, but a misunderstanding of God. It seems pious to neglect our bodies because we are afraid of what that might lead to—or because we simply don't want to sacrifice and put in the work. That's a selfish and lazy attitude based in fear rather than hope. It's like saying you'd rather remain in debt because you're afraid you would misuse wealth or because you just don't want the "restriction" of living on a budget. If we are afraid of what we will become or do with God-given resources, we are telling God, "I hid it because I don't trust your heart. I think you're a hard man, and I was afraid."

What if, instead of looking at the potential risk, we focused on the potential reward. What if you disciplined your body, became healthy and fit, and increased your years of usefulness to the kingdom? What if the changes you make could give the Lord a return on His investment? How much more good could you do? How many more people could you serve? How many could be led to Christ?

The warning to the church is clear. While some are serving the Master and are ready for His return, others are just going through the motions—appearing to serve Him. But true faith produces results, while lack of faith produces nothing. Knowing that we will one day give an account for *everything* should move us to glorify God in everything we do with our bodies and to call on His strength to help us accomplish what He calls us to.

We have been given so much access to good food and clean water. We have the ability and numerous options to exercise. There is so much we know about properly caring for ourselves. And we know, "Everyone to whom much was given, of him much will be required, and from him to whom they entrusted much, they will demand the more" (Luke 12:48 ESV)

Which brings me back to my original question: If you could do better, should you?

The good news is that in Christ you have the power to experience change—deep, fundamental change. It is possible to become tenderhearted when once you were callous and insensitive. It is possible to stop being dominated by bitterness and anger. It is possible to become a loving person no matter what your background has been. And it is possible for a couch potato and glutton (like I was) to become a model of health and fitness—and even a health coach.

The Bible assumes that God is the decisive factor in making us what we should be. Paul said, "And I am sure of this, that he who began a good work in you will bring it to completion at the day of Jesus Christ" (Philippians 1:6 ESV).

Lord command what you will and grant what you command![14]
        —SAINT AUGUSTINE

CHAPTER 5

STRENGTH AND BEAUTY

Splendor and majesty are before him; strength and beauty are in his sanctuary.
>—KING DAVID (Psalms 96:6 ESV)

Beauty is essential to God. No—that's not putting it strongly enough. Beauty is the essence of God.[1]
>—JOHN & STASI ELDREDGE

Beauty is indeed a good gift of God.[2]
>—SAINT AUGUSTINE

She dresses herself with strength and makes her arms strong.
>—KING SOLOMON (Proverbs 31:17 ESV)

Blessed be the Lord, my rock, who trains my hands for war, and my fingers for battle.
>—KING DAVID (Psalms 144:1 ESV)

To be perfectly honest, this chapter came as a complete surprise to me. I had no intention of writing it. In the nine years I have been writing about biblical health and fitness, I have not once taught or written on the idea that our desire to be attractive and physically strong are good things. It's something I have shied away from. So, why now? Because God brought it up.

As I was working on this book, I also was working with a mentor, Denise Needham. Denise is a very dear friend of our family and an amazing woman of God. We first met her in 2009 when she was the Senior Director of Field Development for a fitness company we were partnering with. We had the opportunity to work with her directly on several occasions and developed a lasting friendship.

After Denise left that company, she began a consulting business, and Tracy was in a year-long women's mentorship group that Denise led. Over the years, we had talked with Denise on several occasions about the relationship between faith and fitness and all that the Bible teaches about health. Eventually, we talked with Denise about how God was leading us to really invest into this ministry and to finally write this book. She offered to walk with us through the journey. It was her ministry to us.

So, Denise and I began having weekly video conference calls and we talked and texted throughout the week. A few days before I started writing this chapter, she shared something with me.

"You know what," she said. "In the past couple of months since I have been working with you I have really come to realize that our primary goal for eating clean and working out is to glorify God in our bodies."

Absolutely, I thought to myself.

"But an interesting thing has happened," she continued. "When I stopped thinking about how my decisions affected my weight or my appearance and only thought about it in terms of my relationship with God, I started giving in to temptation. I would think, 'God won't mind if I have this brownie,' and I began to indulge more. Deryl, I've gained fifteen pounds. I was more motivated to stay on track when I was more focused on my appearance."

Interesting, I thought as I confessed to her that I have had the same struggle recently.

Ok, God, what's up? What have I missed?

I had the opportunity to attend one of Tony Horton's Fitness Camps in July of 2008. You probably know Tony as the creator of P90X®, which is how I was first introduced to him. I had already had the pleasure of meeting Tony on a couple of occasions, including when I was flown to Los Angeles for an infomercial shoot with him.

If you have seen the infomercials or done the workouts, you know that Tony is a bit of a comedian—and that he loves to show off his abs and biceps. Of course, if you were in that kind of shape at any age (especially in your 50's), I'm willing to bet you would be proud of yours too. But when it comes to health and fitness, Tony is quite serious.

I learned so much at that Fitness Camp. That was where I first heard about Dr. John J. Ratey's book, *Spark*, which explains how exercise does as much, if not more, for your brain than for your body. We also heard from Tony's personal chef, Melissa Costello, who shared so much about the power of food to heal the body. But my biggest takeaway came from a reality check that Tony gave us. In a nutshell, he said that most people when they began a workout program are motivated by of vanity. They see an advertisement or watch an infomercial and see all of the success stories—complete with beautiful people with perfect bodies running on the beach. And they want it.

Tony pointed out that fitness companies know this. It's smart advertising. But he also reminded us that wanting to look good isn't a deep enough motivation. Vanity for vanity's sake won't get you past your first real hurdle. People need a deeper reason to stay on track with their workouts and diets.

That, Tony said, is why it's so important to connect with someone who can help you figure out your deeper "why"—that motivation that goes beyond vanity. It might be living better and living longer. It might be eating in a way that nourishes and heals your body each day. It might be making yourself less prone to illness and injury by working to improve your fitness every day, even when you don't feel like it or it's not convenient.

In a word, his thoughts were genius! Yes, everyone wants to look their best. It seems to be hardwired into our mental and emotional DNA. At her core, every woman wants to know that she is beautiful—captivating. At his core, every man wants to know that he is strong—a valiant and dashing warrior. These desires have been in our hearts from Creation. Therefore, they must be part of God's design. These desires only get us into trouble when we seek to fulfill them outside of God's design.

When I first began my transformation, I really was focused on my health. I wanted to live longer. I wanted to live better. But, I wanted to *look* better too.

If we're honest, we all do. As the weight began to come off, and especially as I began really push myself, I began seeing a new reality. I began believing it was possible to get "ripped" for the first time in my life. (I had never had six-pack abs, not even when I had been "thin.") I began thinking it was possible for me to do more than a couple of pull-ups. I was becoming increasingly strong and vibrant and confident.

Can I be real for a moment? It also felt good to turn heads. To be acknowledged for the hard work I had put in. Yes, that can become dangerous. Yes, it can become an idol. But at its core, that desire flows from the image of God in us—not from our fallen nature. The Enemy takes the good gifts of God and twists them, offering us back a pale substitute.

Allow me to explain. In itself, desire is not a bad thing. The belief that desire is bad and must be killed is the lie of the enemy. It is part of his attempt to kill you by killing your soul. As C.S. Lewis said, "If there lurks in most modern minds the notion that to desire our own good and earnestly to hope for the enjoyment of it is a bad thing, I submit that this notion has crept in from Kant and the Stoics and is no part of the Christian faith."[3]

What God tells us through His Word is that He is the author of our deepest desires and that it's His desire to see them fulfilled. King David, writing under the inspiration of the Holy Spirit, said, "Delight yourself in the LORD, and he will give you the desires of your heart" (Psalm 37:4 ESV).

The desires we've held in our hearts since childhood and the deep longings we have even now as adults remind us of the life God intended for us. They reveal what it means to be fully alive. What are these desires? The best and most concise answer I have found came from writer John Eldredge.

As a man, one of the most profound books I have read is Eldredge's *Wild at Heart*. I cannot begin to express the number of ways this book has revealed my true heart and set me free to be a man of God in the truest sense of the words. Regarding the desires of a man's heart, he wrote:

> God meant something when he meant man, and if we are to ever find ourselves we must find that. . . . There are three desires I find written so deeply into my heart I know now I can no longer disregard them without losing my soul. They are core to who and what I am and yearn to be. I gaze into boyhood, I search the pages of Scripture, of literature, I listen carefully to many, many men, and I am convinced these desires are universal, a clue into masculinity itself. They may be misplaced, forgotten, or misdirected, but in the heart of every man is a desperate desire for a battle to fight, an adventure to live, and a beauty to rescue. I want you to think of the films men love, the things they do with their free time, and especially the aspirations of little boys and see if I am not right on this.[4]

At the core, every man's desire is to know that he is strong. As Eldredge points out, "little boys yearn to know they are powerful, they are dangerous, they are someone to be reckoned with."[5] The warrior heart of a man is the image of God in him. "The LORD is a warrior; the LORD is His name" (Exodus 15:3 NASB). The desire for an adventure is also rooted in how we bear the image of God. Adventure is not about being an "adrenaline junkie." It's not all about fun and games. Adventure *requires* something of us. It forces us to be strong and resourceful and courageous.

Even our desire for a beauty to rescue reveals our desire to be strong. That's not because women are weak and need us to rescue them, but it's because they inspire us to be our best. There is nothing in the world as inspiring to a man as a beautiful woman. Women motivate and inspire us to be our best, to show our strength, to be the hero. As Jack Nicholson says to Helen Hunt at the end of *As Good As It Gets,* "You make me want to be a better man."

Men yearn to be strong, not just for themselves, but also for someone in particular. There is a scene in *The Lion, the Witch, and the Wardrobe* where Susan, the eldest sister and second eldest of the four Pevensie children is about to meet Aslan, a Lion who rules over Narnia and serves as the Christ-figure in the series, for the first time. Once Susan discovers Aslan is a lion, she asks her friend, Mr. Beaver, if he is "quite safe." Beaver explains that Aslan is not safe at all—but he is good. And he is king.[6]

That is the desire of man's heart—to be strong and dangerous and rugged and good.

That's who Jesus was. He was meek—He demonstrated strength under control. That doesn't mean that He was a weakling or a pushover. He turned over tables and drove the money-changing thieves out of the Temple. He walked right through the middle of a crowd that was ready to throw Him off a cliff. He stood against evil and refused to follow meaningless traditions—even if it rubbed religious leaders the wrong way.

That's not a "nice" guy. That's someone you don't want to mess with. But He was also infinitely and completely good.

Are you following? It seems almost counter-intuitive, right? There is something oddly paradoxical in the combination of strength and gentleness in the essence of a godly man.

Don't worry ladies, I haven't forgotten about you. There is a companion book to *Wild at Heart,* written by John and his wife, Stasi, called *Captivating.* Just as I encourage every man I talk with to read *Wild at Heart,* I encourage women to read *Captivating* to find the understanding and freedom they need to become the women they were created to be. While each book focuses primarily on speaking to men or women, respectively, both give readers a glimpse into the heart and soul of the other. In *Wild at Heart,* John speaks profoundly to the heart of women:

> There are also three desires that I have found essential to a woman's heart, which are not entirely different from a man's and yet they remain distinctly feminine. Not every woman wants a battle to fight, but every woman yearns to be fought for. Listen to the longing of a woman's heart: she wants to be more than noticed—she wants to be wanted. She wants to be pursued.
>
>   Every woman also wants an adventure to share. . . . To be cherished, pursued, fought for—yes. But also, . . . to be strong and a part of the adventure. . . . A woman doesn't want to be the

adventure; she wants to be caught up into something greater than herself.

And finally, every woman wants to have a beauty to unveil. Not to conjure, but to unveil. Most women feel the pressure to be beautiful from very young, but that is not what I speak of. There is also a deep desire to simply and truly be the beauty, and be delighted in.[7]

Angela Thomas also uses this quote in her book, *Do You Think I'm Beautiful?: The Question Every Woman Asks*. Her reaction as a woman to his words is:

Wow, he gets it. This guy has listened past the surface of women and heard them ask the questions:
Who will fight for me?
Who will be my hero?
Who will call me beautiful?
I cried over these words because Eldredge doesn't seem to hold the questions against us. He can see that they are legitimately woven into the core of every woman's soul. He reminds us that we cannot get to the answers that heal and restore until we have asked the questions that penetrate our hidden desires.[8]

So why do we have such a hard time grasping the essential nature of beauty? Why do Christians, well-meaning men and women, seek to minimize, or worse, dismiss it? Perhaps we have the words of Proverbs 31:30 in our minds: "Charm is deceitful, and beauty is vain, but a woman who fears the LORD is to be praised" (Proverbs 31:30 ESV). But let's break this down. Is it really saying that women should not be charming or beautiful? Hardly, since those are attributes that are praised elsewhere. King Solomon, gifted by God with a heart of wisdom, extols the beauty, allure and gracefulness of his beloved throughout the Song of Songs—a beautiful and at times very sensual poetic book. How interesting that within the canon of Scripture, God provides us with an expression of romantic love between a man and woman.

I believe the key to understanding Proverbs 31 lies in what the writer saw as the highest attribute. No matter how flattering, alluring and beautiful a woman is, none of those qualities really cover up an ill-natured, bitter, quarrelsome, depraved spirit. And no beauty is worth putting up with that. As another writer in Proverbs said, "It is better to live in a desert land than with a contentious and vexing woman" (Proverbs 21:19 NASB).

Outward beauty, by itself, is nothing. It is worthless. It is vanity. But outward beauty that flows from—and is magnified by—inner beauty, now that is something! That is the nature of God reflected in a woman's life.

God is Himself beautiful. In the words of John and Stasi Eldredge, "Beauty is essential to God—no that's not putting it strongly enough. Beauty is the essence of God."[9] John Piper proclaimed, "From eternity to eternity, the beauty of God is pervasive and practical."[10] Actually, *beautiful* doesn't even begin to describe Him. We have no words that do Him justice, only a deep longing to behold His beauty. As David sang, "One thing have I asked of the LORD, that will I seek after: that I may dwell in the house of the Lord all the days of my life, *to gaze upon the beauty of the LORD* and to inquire in his temple" (Psalm 27:4 ESV, *emphasis mine*).

Not only is God the very definition of beauty, but He also delights in beauty. As Genesis declares, "God saw all that He had made, and behold, it was very good" (Genesis 1:31 NASB). While most English translations render the Hebrew *tov* as "good" in this verse, the Septuagint—the Greek translation of the Old Testament—used the word for "beautiful" (*kalos*) instead of "good" (*agathos*).

Speaking of songs and beauty, I am deeply moved by music. It is powerful beyond words. I can hear the instrumental of *O Holy Night* and be moved to tears as my heart sings the words. Then again, I am a musician. There are moments when I am playing with a worship team that it is all I can do to keep playing because I am so overwhelmed by the beauty and grace of God.

There is a song called, *Spirit Move* on the Bethel album, *Have It All* (Do they still call them albums or am I just showing my age?). The chorus is a call to pursue one thing: to know God and see His beauty—the same plea King David made, "*to gaze upon the beauty of the LORD.*"

Yes and Amen!!

There is beauty in music. Psalm 33:3 says, "Sing to Him a new song; Play skillfully with a shout of joy" (NASB). One translation renders it "Sing a new song to him. Play beautifully and joyfully on stringed instruments" (GWT). The verb translated "skillfully" is from the Hebrew root that means "to be good, well, glad, or pleasing." Once again, the Septuagint translators chooses *kalos* or "beautiful" when they got to this word. When combined with the verb for playing instruments the idea is to play skillfully, expertly—beautifully. It's a reminder that we're to "use well" the gifts God provides. In the case of musical talent, playing skillfully and beautifully requires years of dedication, commitment and diligent practice. It challenges us to work hard to make the most of the gifts we've been given—and to offer them back to the Lord joyfully.

It is a joyful commitment to excellence.

Now for the parallel. When you watch a worship team and hear artists who have worked long and hard to perfect their craft play something that stirs your soul, do you think to yourself, *Look at how arrogant and vain they are. Look at how much fun they are having. This is all about them and how good they are. Think of all of the hours they wasted practicing. They could have used that time to better serve God.* Of course not! That's ridiculous. They are serving God. So, why would you look at a brother or sister in Christ, who understands that their body belongs to God and is a thing of beauty meant to glorify Him, with a critical eye? Why would you look at believers who have dedicated themselves and disciplined their body to bring it into submission with contempt and judge them as vain and selfish people?

People who are healthy and physically fit tend to radiate joy. They tend to glow. They tend to be happier. They tend to be the most beautiful version of themselves inside and out. And that's not a bad thing!

Everything God creates is beautiful. David exalts, "The heavens declare the glory of God" (Psalms 19:1 ESV); and Isaiah wrote, "The whole earth is full of His glory" (Isaiah 6:3 NASB). How does creation display the glory of God? Primarily through its beauty.

Picture the beauty of a sunset, the majesty of the mountains, or the power of the ocean. Their beauty takes our breath away. One of the most profound experiences of this for me was during my first mission trip to India. We were up in the Himalayas, in the region of Ladakh. We spent the first three days in the capital city of Leh to acclimate to the altitude and then set out trekking through the villages. The first night out, we set up camp in a village that probably sat somewhere around 13,000 feet above sea level. After hiking through the hauntingly beautiful Himalayas during the day, I looked up that night into a sky with no light pollution. More than two miles above sea level, what I saw literally took my breath away. I hit my knees and wept at the beauty of the heavens and the beauty of the One who created them—and yet still cared for me. That is probably the closest I will ever come to what Isaiah experienced when he saw the glory of the Lord and proclaimed, "Woe is me, for I am undone!"(Isaiah 6:5 NKJV). And all I saw was the beauty God created in nature. As Eldredge said, "Nature is not primarily functional. It is primarily beautiful."[11] God is both beautiful and delights in beauty.

The reason a woman desires to know that she is beautiful, that she is captivating, is because that is the part of the image of God knitted into her being, it is her essence. She wants her beauty—both internal and external— to be revealed and recognized because God does. If a woman's beauty is measured only by whether or not she has a flat stomach or defined legs or pleasing features or any other physical attribute, then we are lost. True beauty is the combination of *both* outward physical beauty and inner spiritual/soulful beauty. We cannot allow the world's perversion of beauty to rob us of the ability to appreciate godly beauty.

> Yes, the world cheapens and prostitutes beauty, making at all about a perfect figure few women can attain. But Christians minimize it too, or overspiritualize it, making it all about "character." We must recover the prize of Beauty. The church must take it back. Beauty is too vital to lose. God gave Eve a beautiful form *and* a beautiful spirit. She expresses beauty in both. Better, she expresses beauty simply in who she is. Like God, it is her *essence*.[12]

Strength and beauty are part of how men and women bear the image of God. God is a warrior. Man is a warrior. God is beautiful. Woman is beautiful. Ultimately, we bear the image of God to point others to Him. As. C.S. Lewis said, "We do not want to merely "see" beauty—though, God knows, even that is bounty enough. We want something else which can hardly be put into words–to be united with the beauty we see, to pass into it, to receive it into ourselves, to bathe in it, to become part of it."[13]

We catch but a glimpse of that here on earth, but one day we will know and experience Beauty fully. That eternal day is coming. In the meantime, we are God's image bearers.

How we take care of our bodies directly affects how well we reveal the image of God in us. Like it or not, we judge each other by how we take care of ourselves. When we see someone who is physically fit, a part of us recognizes the discipline and dedication it takes to achieve that, especially in a culture that does everything it can to sabotage our health. We respect that. Likewise, right or wrong, when we see an obese person, our first thought is often that they are lazy and undisciplined.

Recently I was talking with one of our campus ministers and he said, "Have you ever heard a preacher speak who was obese and automatically disregard what they are saying? I have." I have too. Even when I was overweight myself. I think that's part of what Paul meant when he said, "But I discipline my body and keep it under control, lest after preaching to others I myself should be disqualified" (1 Corinthians 9:27 ESV).

It's also a documented fact that our fitness level affects our paycheck. On weight-based discrimination in the workplace, personal financial expert Carmen Wong Ulrich said:

Wage discrimination exists as well as hiring discrimination. The majority of respondents in one recent study said that they'd always choose the thinner individual when deciding between two similar job applicants. Employees who are overweight, on average, make $1.25 an hour less than a low-BMI colleague, adding up to a six-figure loss over a career. Women get hit the hardest when it comes to paying a high price at work for being overweight — obese women can make up to 24 percent less than an average-size women while even slightly overweight women make around 6 percent less.[14]

We are attracted to strength and beauty. The desire to be strong and beautiful is innate and God-given. They just can't be our primary motivation. That's what Tony was talking about that day at his fitness camp. If your desire to look better is the motivation that gets you started on your journey to better health, there is absolutely nothing wrong with that—as long as you don't violate God's plan for your health.

What do I mean by that? Whenever I am doing my initial consultation with a client, one question I ask is, "Are you primarily interested in losing weight, or improving your health?" They almost always ask, "What's the difference." It's simple. There are tons of things you can do to lose weight, to get lean and ripped, but not all of them will make you healthier. In fact, some of them will actually increase your risk of illness and injury.

The bodybuilding and fitness competition world is full of examples of this. Contestants put all kinds of artificial ingredients, toxins, and poisons into their bodies in the form of "health" supplements (more on that later). Walk into many "health" or "nutrition" stores and most of the supplements you find on the shelves should never find their way into your body. People drive themselves crazy with super-strict, repetitive bland meal plans, all to maximize fat-burning. They dehydrate themselves and do whatever else it takes to get to that "look" to win the competition or to be ready for the photo shoot. A friend who competes in bodybuilding competitions told me that bodybuilders are at their weakest on competition day.

It's crazy. Even worse, it's unhealthy.

If that's what you want, this is not the book for you. You need to find somebody else to be your coach. When I work with clients, we focus on living a healthy lifestyle. When you do the things that give you optimal health (love God, love others, eat clean, train hard, live with passion and purpose…) then you will have the optimal body for you. You will be your best. You will be your strongest and your most beautiful, without having to compare yourself to anybody else. And when you master the discipline of being physically fit and healthy, you can master anything.

Discipline is a lot like a muscle. The more you use it, the easier other things become. You find you can be more disciplined with your time with God. You find that when you are healthy you tend to be in a better mood. You tend to be more stable. Your brain functions better. You become the best version of you possible. And that is a beautiful thing.

THE FOUNTAIN OF YOUTH

[God] has planted eternity in the human heart.
        —KING SOLOMON (Ecclesiastes 3:11, NLT)

"Bless the LORD, O my soul . . . who satisfies you with good so that your youth is renewed like the eagle's."
        —KING DAVID (Psalms 103:1,5 ESV)

Aging is for people who don't know better.
        —TONY HORTON

There is something within the human heart that knows we were meant to live forever. Solomon, who famously said that there is a time to live and a time to die (Ecclesiastes 3:2), also said that God has planted eternity in the human heart (Ecclesiastes 3:11). I believe it's another one of those impressions pressed into the memory of our DNA—the memory that our first parents were created in a Garden and were designed to live forever. And they would have if it had not been for The Fall. It was God's mercy that forced Adam and Eve out of the Garden and blocked the way "lest [they] reach out [their] hand and take also of the tree of life and eat, and live forever" (Genesis 3:22 ESV).

But that desire for eternal youth, beauty and perfection still lingers because it is why we were originally created—and it is our ultimate destination. In the meantime, we're caught in a longing for what will be revealed (Romans 8:19). I believe that is why the quest for eternal youth— a way to stay forever young—has consumed the hearts and minds of human beings throughout history. For thousands of years of recorded history, across a variety of cultures and people groups, there have been stories of a magical "fountain of youth." In the 5th century B.C., the Greek historian Herodotus wrote about a fountain in the land of the Macrobians that gave the people exceptionally long life and youthfulness.[15] Stories like this can be found throughout history and culture right up to the fabled "Fountain of Youth" for which Ponce de Leon allegedly searched in Florida. As many retirees as there are moving to Florida to live out their years, you'd think many are still looking for it. I used to live in Florida. We still vacation there. From the look of things, they haven't found it yet.

Nope, nobody gets out of this life alive. Everyone grows old. Everyone eventually dies. Of course, Jesus will return for His people and those of us who are around will be caught up in the rapture (a trip I am beginning to think this generation has a pretty good chance of making), but that's a different story. In general, our days are numbered.

Do you know what that number is? It's actually relative. In the United States, for example, the average life expectancy is 79.3 years (81.6 years for women, 76.9 years for men). Would it surprise you to know that the U.S. ranks 31st in the world in life expectancy? Yep, we're definitely doing something wrong here.

Japan is ranked first, with an average life expectancy of 83.7 years. They get four more years. That's an average mind you, which means there are people who live longer—and some lives are much shorter.

Care to know what the oldest recorded age for a human is? One woman lived 122 years. Her name was Jeanne Louise Calment. She was born on February 21, 1875, and died on August 4, 1997. That's 122 years, 164 days old. This is referred to as the maximum life span, the upper boundary of life, the maximum number of years a human can live. Hsu Yun, a Chinese Buddhist master, lived to be 119 years old. He was born in 1840 and died in 1959. These may seem like extreme examples, but they are nothing compared to what we find in the first chapters of Genesis. Prior to The Flood men lived centuries, not decades. Adam lived 930 years. Methuselah, who lived to the age of 969, is the oldest person in the biblical records. Noah lived to be 950.

After the Flood things started to change: "Then the LORD said, "My Spirit shall not abide in man forever, for he is flesh: his days shall be 120 years" (Genesis 6:3 ESV). From Noah to Moses, we see a gradual decline in life spans to around 120 years.

If God set our life span at 120 years, why does our average fall so short of that? Why are people like Jeanne Calment and Hsu Yun the exception? Why are we losing a full third of our years? Maybe it's because we are killing ourselves.

When I talk about wanting to live to 100 to 120 years, people look at me like I'm crazy. I get reactions like, "I would never want to live that long? Who wants to suffer the ravages of age that long?" Indeed. But who said anything about spending 40 years hunched over and barely able to move. That's not life. But what if you could *live* for 120 years and be active? What if you could be productive and enjoy time with your loved ones? What if you could make a difference in the world—like Moses did?

There may not be a Fountain of Youth, but you have a lot to say about what your last years look like. When I see elderly people hunched over, crippled by arthritis, shuffling around (if they can even walk), or worse trapped in a bed having someone else turn them to prevent bed sores, it breaks my heart. To see the cares and pains of life etched into their faces, to watch them stare out the windows of a nursing home at a world they can no longer enjoy, it makes me want to weep.

And it's not just the elderly. Men and women in their 40's and 50's are ravaged by the effects of diabetes, heart disease, or cancer. Children of God, created in His image, can barely get around and are living in constant pain. This is not what God intended.

We know this because we see the exceptions to what has become the rule. We talk about these diseases and illnesses, along with the loss of mobility, strength, and freedom as the natural process of aging; but, as Tony Horton said, "Aging is for people who don't know better!"[16]

I know people, men and women in their 70's and 80's, who are still active every day. They have the look and mobility of someone decades younger. The difference is in their choices. They walk, and they play. They even do push-ups! They eat foods that are amazingly delicious and life-giving. You can make the same choices. It's not too late for you. It's never too late—until it is.

According to Dr. C. Norman Shealy, Tony is on to something. The average life expectancy in the United States is now 79 years. But who wants to be just average? Not me. In his book *Life Beyond 100*, Dr. Shealy says if you're a non-smoker you can add six years. If you maintain a reasonable weight, you can add six years. If you exercise regularly, you can add six years. If your average alcohol intake is one drink per day or less, you can add three years. If you avoid street drugs, you can add two years. According to Dr. Shealy's research, if you just do those few very simple things, you can add 23 years to your life expectancy. Now you're up to 102.

Anybody interested in adding a couple of productive, fulfilling decades to your life?

Would it surprise you to learn that not everybody finds that appealing? Sometimes when I talk about wanting to be a centenarian, I hear something along the lines of "I don't want to wait that long to get to Heaven." OK. I understand that one. But it's a bit selfish, don't you think? God has set eternity in our hearts. As Paul said, "to live is Christ, but to die is gain" (Philippians 1:21). Of course, we long for heaven, and we will never be fully satisfied until we reach that eternal country. That is our future. That is our ultimate hope. Nothing we accomplish here on earth will ever begin to compare. But we cannot be so heavenly minded that we are no earthly good. That's why Paul said to live *is* Christ.

As the song *Great Are You Lord* reminds us, it is His breath in our lungs, therefore we praise Him—we offer Him our lives. The way we live our lives should point people to Jesus—our lives are to be a "living sacrifice" right here, right now. Yes, our final destination is Paradise; but God, who has known us from before time, has a purpose and a plan for our lives in the present.

My life verse is Ephesians 2:10. It says, "For we are his workmanship, created in Christ Jesus for good works, which God prepared beforehand, that we should walk in them." (Ephesians 2:10 ESV). We are masterpieces—like the Sistine Chapel! We are new creations—reborn, renewed, set apart and empowered—set aside to be His hands and feet. All we have to do is act on His work in our lives!

According to this verse, we were created for life in both this age and the age to come. Earth may not be our final home, but there can and should be joy in the journey to heaven. As Solomon wisely said, "I perceived that there is nothing better for them than to be joyful and to do good as long as they live" (Ecclesiastes 3:12 ESV). This life is the proving ground for the next. We should be fully alive in this life. We should prosper where God has planted us. Then we will hear the Master say, "Well done, good and faithful servant. Enter now into the joy of your Master" (Matthew 25:21) Then we will be transformed from fully alive to *fully alive*!!

FINDING FREEDOM

I love the writing of C.S. Lewis. I have read the entire *Chronicles of Narnia* series several times throughout my life. Every book in the series is absolutely exceptional, and I love them as much as an adult as I ever did as a child—probably more so. C.S. Lewis reveals so many deep truths through allegory that I didn't really understand until I was an adult. I now have the thrill of getting to share these beloved classics with my children. I pray that God uses them to touch their hearts as much as they have mine.

There is a scene in *The Voyage of the Dawn Treader* that—even to this day—rocks me to my core. Over the course of a few pages Lewis gave us one of the most powerfully moving pictures of the grace and mercy of God at work in the process of salvation.

In order to properly understand the scene, we need to know what has led up to this moment. Eustace Clarence Scrubb was a rather rotten boy who discovered a large treasure in a cave. He placed one of the gold bracelets on his arm and fell asleep dreaming of the treasure and what he will do with it. When he woke up he discovered that he had been turned into a dragon. The gold bracelet he put on his arm was now digging into his dragon leg—causing a great deal of pain. The worst part though was when he realized that he was now all alone, unable to communicate or connect with his cousins, the Pevensies, or any other human for that matter. He realizes how horrible he has been and what a burden he now is others. He begins to weep.

Enter Aslan. Aslan is the Christ-figure of the *Chronicles*. He is the King and son of the Emperor across the Sea. He is also a Lion. Aslan has compassion on the boy-turned-dragon, and leads Eustace to a garden on top of a mountain. In the center of the garden is a large round well—so big that it was more like a bath with marble steps going down into it.

Eustace thinks to himself that if he could just get into the water it would ease the pain in his leg. But Aslan told him he must undress first. At first Eustace is confused, but then remembers that dragons, like snakes, can cast off their skins. He begins scratching himself with his dragon claws and scales begin to fall off all around him as his skin started peeling off. In a couple of minutes he is able to step out of it, but as he starts to get into the water, he looks and sees his reflection. Realizing he has another layer of dragon skin, he begins to peel off the second layer. He gets it off only to discover there is another layer. He goes through the process a third time only to realize all of his efforts were in vain—he's still a dragon.

That's when Aslan said, "You will have to let me undress you." Even though Eustace was afraid of Aslan's claws, he was so desperate to get the dragon skin off he laid down on his back and surrendered to Aslan's will. Eustace recounts what happened next to his cousin, Edmund:

> "The very first tear he made was so deep that I thought it had gone right into my heart. And when he began pulling the skin off, it hurt worse than anything I've ever felt. The only thing that made me able to bear it was just the pleasure of feeling the stuff peel off. You know—if you've ever picked the scab of a sore place. It hurts like billy-oh but it is such fun to see it coming away."
>
> "I know exactly what you mean," said Edmund.
>
> "Well, he peeled the beastly stuff right off—just as I thought I'd done it myself the other three times, only they hadn't hurt—and there it was lying on the grass: only ever so much thicker, and darker, and more knobbly looking than the others had been. And there was I as smooth and soft as a peeled switch and smaller than I had been. Then he caught hold of me—I didn't like that much for I was very tender underneath now that I'd no skin on—and threw me into the water. It smarted like anything but only for a moment. After that it became perfectly delicious and as soon as I started swimming and splashing I found that all the pain had gone from my arm. And then I saw why. I'd turned into a boy again. You'd think me simply phoney if I told you how I felt about my own arms. I know they've no muscle and are pretty mouldy compared with Caspian's, but I was so glad to see them.
>
> After a bit the lion took me out and dressed me . . . in new clothes."[1]

The first time I read this story I remember being slightly embarrassed as the tears welled up in my eyes and began to flow down my cheek. I was overcome by emotion as I saw myself in Eustace. I knew my true self was hidden under layers of doubt and fear, hurts and addictions. I knew that when I tried to fix myself by myself, I always fell short. I needed help. I needed Jesus to do what Aslan did—pierce deep enough to remove the layers. I needed Him to cleanse me, clothe me, and set me free.

That's exactly what Jesus offered the church at Laodicea in Revelation 3. It is what he offers us today.

By now, you're probably starting to realize how important our health and fitness are to the heart of God. But knowing is not enough. We must do something about it. As James said, "Don't just listen to God's word. You must do what it says. Otherwise, you are only fooling yourselves" (James 1:22 NLT). Now that you understand why taking care of your body is important, it is time to talk about how you can do that. The slogan I created for Ardent Fitness is: *Eat Clean. Train Hard. Live Passionately!* That's it in a nutshell. Eating clean we sort of understand. Training hard is a relative concept. Living passionately is a little more vague because it incorporates every area of life. It's a great slogan. Short. Concise. True.

For the purpose of teaching and unpacking what each part means and how we live them out, let's think of it like building a house. First, we must lay a strong, unshakeable foundation. In *The Daniel Plan*, Pastor Rick Warren says the first of five essentials is faith. That is followed by food, fitness, focus and friends.[2] I tend to talk about faith, food, fitness, focus, and fellowship because I happen to like "fellowship" better than "friends"—maybe because I'm a *Lord of the Rings* nerd.

Anyway, the bottom line is that when all five essentials are in place, we have something strong enough to support not just our physical health, but a healthy life—an abundant life. Then we will be fully alive.

CHAPTER 6

THE FOUNDATION OF FAITH

"And without faith it is impossible to please [God]"
— (Hebrews 11:6 NASB)

"I can do all things through [Christ] who strengthens me."
—(Philippians 4:13 ESV)

Eustace's story from the last chapter reminds us that deep and lasting change is not possible apart from the power of God in Christ. Willpower alone is never enough—not long term. Sure, we can make small changes. We can even make big changes temporarily. But anything done in our own strength won't last.

Maybe you've experienced this in your life. How many diets have you been on only to gain the weight back? Have you ever made a resolution to start working out and join a gym on January 1? If you're like most people, you go every day for a few weeks and then you miss a workout or two. That stretches to three or four, and the next thing you know you haven't worked up a sweat in weeks—maybe even months or years. Or maybe you set a goal to start having a date night with your spouse at least twice a month. Things start out great and then life happens. (Just so you know . . . I'm talking to myself here too. I'm guilty of all of these!)

But before we start condemning ourselves too harshly, remember that we are in good company. We can agree with Paul that there is a war within us: "I want to do what is right, but I can't. I want to do what is good, but I don't. I don't want to do what is wrong, but I do it anyway" (Rom 7:18–19 NLT).

Every time I read this passage, my heart cries out, *That's me! That's me!* "Wretched man that I am! Who will deliver me from this body of death?" (Romans 7:24 ESV) And just as despair begins to well up in my heart, I cry out with the great Apostle, "Thanks be to God through Jesus Christ our

Lord! So then, I myself serve the law of God with my mind, but with my flesh I serve the law of sin" (Rom 7:25 ESV).

And it gets better!

Paul began one of the greatest chapters in the Bible with these words: "There is therefore now no condemnation for those who are in Christ Jesus" (Rom 8:1 ESV).

I love how Paul explained our brokenness, our life in the Spirit, and how the Father, Son and Spirit work in our lives to bring about certain victory. He reasoned, "What then shall we say to these things? If God is for us, who can be against us?" (Romans 8:31 ESV). As if that wasn't hope enough, he let loose a flurry of rhetorical questions:

> "He who did not spare his own Son but gave him up for us all, how will he not also with him graciously give us all things? Who shall bring any charge against God's elect? It is God who justifies. Who is to condemn? Christ Jesus is the one who died—more than that, who was raised—who is at the right hand of God, who indeed is interceding for us. Who shall separate us from the love of Christ? Shall tribulation, or distress, or persecution, or famine, or nakedness, or danger, or sword?" (Romans 8:32–35 ESV).

And then the grand finale:

> "In all these things we are more than conquerors through him who loved us. For I am sure that neither death nor life, nor angels nor rulers, nor things present nor things to come, nor powers, nor height nor depth, nor anything else in all creation, will be able to separate us from the love of God in Christ Jesus our Lord" (Romans 8:37–39 ESV).

Amen!!! Is it any wonder that this is one of the most beloved chapters in all of Scripture? What a picture it paints of the depths of the Father's love for us—and the power that He works in us through the sacrifice of Christ and intercession of the Holy Spirit!

Is it a sin for us to continue to neglect and abuse our bodies when we know better? Absolutely! Does it affect our salvation or condemn us before God? Absolutely not.

It does however bear consequences. Therefore, our foundation, our trust, must be in the One who alone has the power to accomplish it, the One through whom all things are possible. Our foundation is faith, not because it "sanctifies" our desire to be healthy, but because we're dead if we attempt to build on anything less. Nothing else will hold up under the storms that are coming—and storms are coming.

Think about it—how many times in your life have you failed because you trusted in your own strength instead of placing all of your hope in the all-powerful God. Better yet, what "impossible" feat would you have undertaken if you knew that God was with you, went before you, and protected you from behind? Jesus tells us, "What is impossible with man is possible with God" (Luke 18:27 ESV).

God is our healer. He is our Father. He is Abba—Daddy. He will help you if you ask Him. Jesus once asked, "Which one of you, if his son asks him for bread, will give him a stone? Or if he asks for a fish, will give him a serpent? If you then, who are evil, know how to give good gifts to your children, how much more will your Father who is in heaven give good things to those who ask him!" (Matthew 7:9–11 ESV).

God is a good Father and Creator. He knows us better than we know ourselves. He knows what we need most. If you ask Him to help you improve your health—something He clearly desires for you—He will. His desire is for you to be healthy in spirit, soul, and body.

Remember how we are triune in nature? You are not truly healthy if you neglect any one of the three. Fitness is not just about how you look in a mirror or how many push-ups you can do. Health and fitness encompass every aspect of your life and being. Every area of your body and life affect every other area.

Think about it; If you get in an argument with your kids or spouse on the way to church, does it affect your attitude in worship? If you are stressed out over your finances, does it affect your marriage? That works in reverse too, doesn't it? The only way you can be in optimal physical health is to be spiritually and mentally healthy as well.

We start with spiritual health because it is the foundation, but no one knows your body better than God. He knows best how it operates and how to care for it. And He left instructions for us regarding our bodies in His Word. Does that surprise you? It shouldn't. The Bible is an instruction manual for life. "All Scripture is inspired by God and is useful to teach us what is true and to make us realize what is wrong in our lives. It corrects us when we are wrong and teaches us to do what is right. God uses it to prepare and equip his people to do every good work" (2 Timothy 3:16-17 NLT). Did you catch that, not only does God give us instructions, but He also uses them to prepare us and equip us to do what He calls us to do. He supplies the power. Or as Paul says, "I am sure of this, that he who began a good work in you will bring it to completion at the day of Jesus Christ" (Philippians 1:6 ESV).

Oh, I should mention that it's not always a comfortable process. In fact, more often than not it is uncomfortable. I think that's one of those principles God wove into the fabric of life—the refining process requires heat. God's Word doesn't just instruct us. It also penetrates, exposes, and judges. "For the word of God is alive and active. Sharper than any double-edged sword, it penetrates even to dividing soul and spirit, joints and marrow; it judges the thoughts and attitudes of the heart" (Hebrews 4:12 NIV). It is a precise and powerful surgical instrument.

HOW DEEP THE FATHER'S LOVE

I love the song, "How Deep the Father's Love For Us."

How deep the Father's love for us,
How vast beyond all measure,
That He should give His only Son
To make a wretch His treasure.[1]

It's a powerful song rooted in the simple truth of the most well-known verse in the Bible: "For God so loved the world, that he gave his only Son, that whoever believes in him should not perish but have eternal life" (John 3:16 ESV).

Our deepest need is to know that we are loved unconditionally. In that knowledge, we are safe. In that knowledge, we are empowered. We can endure anything as long as we just know that. That's why Paul prayed for us as he did. More than anything else, he wanted us to grasp how deeply God loves us and to live in the power He provides.

"For this reason," he wrote, "I kneel before the Father, from whom every family in heaven and on earth derives its name. I pray that out of his glorious riches he may strengthen you with power through his Spirit in your inner being, so that Christ may dwell in your hearts through faith. And I pray that you, being rooted and established in love, may have power, together with all the Lord's holy people, to grasp how wide and long and high and deep is the love of Christ, and to know this love that surpasses knowledge—that you may be filled to the measure of all the fullness of God" (Ephesians 3:14-19 NIV).

Now that's good stuff! Doesn't that just warm your heart and give you confidence and boldness?

If you want lasting change in your life, if you want the strength to create new life-long, life-giving habits, you must first know the One who gave you life and loves you more than you could ever imagine. The power we have through Him can overcome any obstacle and free you from any bondage.

There is a powerful song that I am sure you have heard in at least one of its versions. Originally written by Will Reagan and performed by Will Reagan and the United Pursuit ban in 2009. It was covered by Jesus Culture in 2011 (That's the version I was most familiar with). In 2012 Gospel singer Tasha Cobbs released her interpretation of the song. Of the three, her YouTube video has the most views. But the version I loved the most was performed on the TV Show *The Voice* by Paxton Ingram in 2016. His performance was so deeply emotional and stirring that the packed house erupted in screams and applause. It was praise—not just for the performance of an individual who dared to share his faith on a secular show, but also for the chain-breaking God he serves. By now you probably know what song I'm talking about: "Break Every Chain."

There is another song I love called "Chain-Breaker," by Zach Williams, that has been getting a lot of airplay on Christian music stations recently. You might just think I'm in some kind of "song mode," but the power of God to free us from the chains that bind us is a theme that touches the deepest places of the human heart. Maybe that's why people write so many songs about it. Or maybe it's because I tend to listen to worship songs while I'm writing. Whatever the reason, the truth remains that the power of God to save and rescue and heal is the inspiration behind some of the most beloved songs in history.

Jesus came "to proclaim that captives will be released, that the blind will see, that the oppressed will be set free" (Luke 4:18 NLT). There is nothing you'll go through that He doesn't already know and understand. There is no temptation you'll face that He hasn't experienced. He's been where you are. The author of Hebrews reminded us, "we do not have a high priest who is unable to sympathize with our weaknesses, but one who in every respect has been tempted as we are, yet without sin" (Hebrews 4:15 ESV). He is our help and our hope.

GOD'S POWER AT WORK IN US

"For it is God who works in you, both to will and to work for his good pleasure."
— (Philippians 2:13 ESV)

Have you struggled to change your health habits in the past? Have you gone on diet after diet—losing weight only to gain it back? Have you promised yourself you will start going to the gym or walking every day only to fall back into your old habits? You may have resigned yourself to believing that you can't change.

I've had people give me the excuse, "You can't teach an old dog new tricks." I don't know where that saying came from, but it's a lie—at least when it comes to humans. Left to your own strength and ability, this is true, but I remind you again that Jesus says, "What is impossible with man is possible with God!" (Luke 18:27 ESV).

Now, even though it is the power of God that works in us, He will not work in us without our cooperation. Think of it like a light switch in your house: God supplies the power and the resources for change, but you must decide and act. If you don't walk over and flip the switch, the light will stay off. You have to change the bulb from time to time. Paul put it like this: "Dear friends, you always followed my instructions when I was with you. And now that I am away, it is even more important. Work hard to show the results of your salvation, obeying God with deep reverence and fear. For God is working in you, giving you the desire and the power to do what pleases him" (Philippians 2:12-13 NLT).

Notice he said both "work hard" (a command for us to do our part to the best of our ability) and "God is working in you" (evidence that He is involved in the process). Both are necessary for change and growth. Notice that it says our hard work reveals "the results of [our] salvation." Hard work is evidence of salvation, not how we earn it. Salvation can neither be earned nor maintained. It is a free gift. God gives it freely and He preserves it: "For it is by grace you have been saved, through faith—and this is not from yourselves, it is the gift of God—not by works, so that no one can boast" (Ephesians 2:8-9 NIV). What sets the Gospel apart from every other religious message in the world is that it's not about what we do to earn God's favor, but what He has done to rescue us. Even the faith that saves us is ultimately a gift from Him.

Part of my motto for Ardent Fitness is *Train Hard*. Admittedly, "hard" is a relative concept. What is hard for an Olympic athlete and what is hard for my five-year-old daughter are two different things. But the point is to push yourself to your limit. When you exercise, you are using muscles that God has given you. As a result, they grow and become stronger. See, fitness is a microcosm of life. The truths and principles apply universally.

There is another parallel between salvation and fitness—both require repentance. Repentance means that we reverse the way we think about something. It's a change of direction. That being said, we won't get it right all of the time. Repentance does not equal perfection. We "are being transformed into His image with ever-increasing glory," (2 Corinthians 3:18 NIV), but it is not a straight shot up. No growth chart is. There are ups and downs along the way, but we maintain a general upward trajectory. As Paul said, "Not that I have already obtained this or am already perfect, but I press on to make it my own, because Christ Jesus has made me his own" (Philippians 3:12 ESV).

When it comes to improving your health and fitness, the first thing you have to do is repent of old ways of thinking, ways that don't serve you. You have to learn to see things the way God sees them, and the best way to do that is through His Word. Paul told us in 2 Timothy, "All Scripture is breathed out by God" (2 Timothy 3:16, ESV). Just like God breathed life into Adam, He breathes life into us through Scripture. The way we repent is to exhale—breathe out—all our old thoughts and attitudes and inhale—breathe in—His Word. Isn't that what Romans 12:2 says? "Don't copy the behavior and customs of this world, but let God transform you into a new person by changing the way you think" (NLT).

As you allow God's Word to change the way you think, He begins to transform you into a new person with new desires. And when you change the way you think and feel about certain things, it changes the way you act. As your actions change, your results change. Or put another way:

"Watch your thoughts, they become words;
watch your words, they become actions;
watch your actions, they become habits;
watch your habits, they become character;
watch your character, for it becomes your destiny."[2]

The only way I know to do this effectively is to stay as close to God as possible. You'll have to exercise your spiritual muscles by committing to the spiritual disciplines of spending time reading God's Word every day, studying it, meditating on it, praying about it, and allowing it to transform you. I cannot emphasize enough how important this is to every area of your life. God is your source of power. Why would you attempt anything without Him?

If you are serious about improving your health and fitness, about improving your life, this is a non-negotiable. If this is a new habit for you, start with 5-10 minutes a day. I also recommend that you start to journal. Write down what God is teaching you, how you are feeling, and observations from Scriptures. Then, talk to God about it in prayer. There is something powerful and transformational about the process of physically writing your thoughts and prayers down with pen and paper.

I promise, you will be amazed at what God does in you through this process.

AN EVER PRESENT HELP

God is our refuge and strength, an ever-present help in trouble.
—(Psalm 46:1 NIV)

This is not going to be easy. It's worth it—well worth it—but it is not easy. Let's just go ahead and get that settled now. You will face trials. You will face temptations. You will fail from time to time. There will be tears of both joy and pain. I have experienced all of these in my fitness journey. I have also experienced all of them as a father. And as a husband. And as a provider for my family. And I wouldn't trade any of it.

In the 1989 movie *Parenthood*, Steve Martin played Gil, the father of the family. In one scene, Gil has been complaining about his complicated life and the trials of parenthood when the Grandma wanders into the room. Grandma tells Gil that when she was nineteen, Grandpa took her on a roller coaster. She goes on to describe how it went up and down, up and down, and what a great ride it was. Gil looks at her like she's lost her marbles and sarcastically comments what a great story it was. Then Grandma showed her wisdom. She said it was so interesting that a ride could make her so frightened and sick and excited and thrilled all at once. Some people don't like roller coasters. They prefer the merry-go-round instead. But that just goes around. It's boring. She likes the roller coaster better—you get more out of it.

Grandma was pretty smart. The question is not whether or not you will have trials—you will. The question is what will you do when you encounter them. Will you rely on God who is our refuge and strength, who is always there ready to help?

Paul reminded us, "No temptation has overtaken you except what is common to mankind. And God is faithful; he will not let you be tempted beyond what you can bear. But when you are tempted, he will also provide a way out so that you can endure it" (1 Corinthians 10:13 NIV). He's also given us His Holy Spirit to work in us and help us when we're weak (Romans 8:26-27).

The apostle John recorded a great word picture that Jesus used to illustrate with Him. He told His disciples, "I am the vine; you are the branches. If you remain in me and I in you, you will bear much fruit; apart from me you can do nothing" (John 15:5 NIV). So, God the Father, God the Holy Spirit, and God the Son are all at work in our lives. Every part of us needs every part of Him.

Don't worry about what happens when you stumble or fall in your journey of health and fitness. Don't worry about the storms that will come.

Remember, you are building your house on the Rock that is Jesus Christ (Matthew 7:24-25). Your house is built on the foundation of faith.

CHAPTER 7

THE PILLAR OF FOOD

So, whether you eat or drink, or whatever you do, do all to the glory of God.
— THE APOSTLE PAUL (1 Corinthians 10:31 ESV)

The food you eat can be either the safest and most powerful form of medicine, or the slowest form of poison.[1]
— DR. ANN WIGMORE, N.D.

In *The Screwtape Letters*, renowned author and Christian apologist C.S. Lewis presents a morally inverted universe that unveils the tactics of the unseen spiritual forces of darkness. Screwtape, a highly placed assistant to "Our Father Below" is writing to his novice demon nephew, Wormwood, and trying to help him draw his assigned patient away from the Enemy (God). As one of Hell's most experienced tempters, Screwtape shares with his nephew the insights he has gained into the heart and foolishness of men. In one case, the "patient" has been experiencing a spiritual "dryness," and Screwtape points out that these periods are an excellent opportunity to appeal to desires for pleasure. Screwtape writes:

Never forget that when we are dealing with any pleasure in its healthy and normal and satisfying form, we are, in a sense, on the Enemy's ground. I know we have won many a soul through pleasure. All the same, it is His invention, not ours. He made the pleasures: all our research so far has not enabled us to produce one. All we can do is to encourage the humans to take the pleasures which our Enemy has produced, at times, or in ways, or in degrees, which He has forbidden. Hence we always try to work away from the natural condition of any pleasure to that in which it is least natural, least redolent of its Maker, and least pleasurable. An ever increasing craving for an ever diminishing pleasure is the formula.

It is more certain; and it's better style. To get the man's soul and give him nothing in return — that is what really gladdens our Father's heart. . . . Talk to him about "moderation in all things". If you can once get him to the point of thinking that "religion is all very well up to a point", you can feel quite happy about his soul. A moderated religion is as good for us as no religion at all — and more amusing.[2]

Pleasure is God's invention. He created us to experience and delight in things that enrapture our senses. That includes food, sex and everything else that is pleasurable. What our enemy does is tempt us to experience his twisted versions of the things that God intended as a blessing. We sacrifice God's best for cheap substitutes—and for what? The enemy deadens our souls, steals our happiness, and destroys our bodies. It's not worth it.

Screwtape's last line always stops me in my tracks—"A moderated religion is as good for us as no religion at all—and more amusing." I have heard this type of reasoning all too often from others and have even been guilty of it myself. We want to put God in a nice little box, tucked away for Sunday mornings or whenever we need Him. Meanwhile, we forget that He is *Lord* of all! We don't own a single area of our lives. Screwtape later writes to Wormwood:

The sense of ownership in general is always to be encouraged. The humans are always putting up claims to ownership which sound equally funny in Heaven and in Hell and we must keep them doing so. . . . And all the time the joke is that the word "Mine" in its fully possessive sense cannot be uttered by a human being about anything. In the long run either Our Father or the Enemy will say "Mine" of each thing that exists, and specially of each man. They will find out in the end, never fear, to whom their time, their souls, and their bodies really belong — certainly not to them, whatever happens.[3]

Over the course of my time in seminary and in talking with pastor friends over the past 10 years, I have often heard that the most "difficult" sermons to preach, in terms of offending your audience, are ones that deal with subjects we tend to claim ownership over. Money and tithing are a common example; but I have told many people that if they think teaching on tithing is hard, they should try teaching on food—especially in the South. Food is one of those subjects that hits painfully close to home, and it reveals the condition of our hearts. I cannot tell you how many times I have had people I love, people I have been in fellowship with, turn on me and accuse me of being a pawn of the devil or teaching "doctrines of demons" because I talk about staying away from certain foods. Generally, it is wrapped within the argument, "Don't tell me what I should or should not eat. It's *my* body, not yours."

Newsflash—it's not your body. But we've already covered that.

In any case, if I had a dime for every time I heard someone tell me that God doesn't care about what they eat or how they'll never give up this or that food or drink, I'd have a mountain of dimes. And every time I hear it, I cringe because it reveals a deeper and much more serious problem than just food. What we are saying is that we are withholding at least one place in our lives from God—a place we think He has no business interfering.

But here's a question: If you owned a million-dollar race horse, how would you take care of it? Would you let him stay up late at night, drink sodas and double mocha lattes, or eat pizza, donuts and fried foods? Would you let him lay around his stall all day watching TV and playing video games? Of course not! Because if you did, he would be become fat, lazy, and completely worthless as a racehorse.

I like that example, and I'm indebted to Zig Ziglar for it. But maybe you prefer horsepower to actual horses. So let's change the scenario. Suppose you were handed the keys to a $200,000 Lamborghini and entrusted with its upkeep. How would you take care of this car? What kind of fuel would you put in it? Regular unleaded? Diesel? Or course not! You would be putting the super premium in this baby. Without the proper fuel, a car like that cannot run at peak performance.

If we would take great care in how we treated a million-dollar race horse or high performance car, shouldn't we take even better care of our bodies which are the temple of the Holy Spirit? Why do we put inferior fuel (food) into these infinitely more valuable marvels of engineering that God has entrusted us with?

All I ask, is that you approach this question like my friend, Sarah, did — with open eyes and an open heart, asking God to reveal His truth to you. As we sat at our breakfast table that morning, I had Sarah open up her Bible and read the passages where God deals with this topic of food. Whenever she had a question about interpretation, I would ask her to read other Scriptures. That's an important thing to do when studying any verse. We have to look at the context. A Bible passage must be understood, not just as it relates to the surrounding text, but also to the whole of Scripture. As social media guru, Gary Vaynerchuk, says: "If content is king, then context is God."[4] Or perhaps you have heard the adage renowned theologian D.A. Carson attributed to his father: "A text without a context is a pretext for a proof text."[5]

already seen from our study of 1 Corinthians 6 that our bodies to God and therefore we should glorify Him in them. Paul reminded us that although all things are lawful, a lot of things aren't good for us. As a result, we should never allow our desires to enslave us. Our God is a jealous God, and He has a zero tolerance policy when it comes to idols. To prove He's serious about that, He used the first two of the Ten Commandments to spell it out for us: "You must not have any other god but me. You must not make for yourself an idol of any kind or an image of anything in the heavens or on the earth or in the sea. You must not bow down to them or worship them, for I, the LORD your God, am a jealous God who will not tolerate your affection for any other gods" (Exodus 20:3-5 NLT). Most of us don't have graven images sitting around our house, but we might have some idols in our hearts. An idol is anything that replaces or supersedes the one, true God.

The Apostle Paul lamented, "For I have told you often before, and I say it again with tears in my eyes, that there are many whose conduct shows they are really enemies of the cross of Christ. They are headed for destruction. Their god is their appetite, they brag about shameful things, and they think only about this life here on earth" (Philippians 3:18-19 NLT). Some translations read, "their god is their belly" (3:19). In a broad sense, "appetite" or "belly" refers to all the physical desires of the flesh, but that certainly includes the stomach and gluttony. In that sense, your god becomes your belly whenever your appetite dictates what you eat and drink regardless of the consequences to your health and the damage it does to your body.

Paul also said that these people glory in their shame. In other words they boast about the wrong that they are doing. When we boast about our large size, our over-eating, how we have built God a bigger temple, or that we will just get to Heaven sooner, we are glorying in our shame. We wink at our sin and cheapen the grace God poured out at Calvary. Paul called such boasters the "enemies of the cross of Christ" and said their "end is destruction." He wasn't being a legalist, and he took no joy in saying these things. On the contrary, he was weeping as he wrote these verses because he knew that these people were only destroying themselves. It broke his heart.

What we put in our bodies should glorify God. We are to serve and love God with all that we are and in everything we do (1 Corinthians 10:31). So, how do we eat and drink to the glory of God? What's that look like?

I used to think that just meant we were supposed to pray over our food and thank God for it. While that's a great idea and we should do it, saying grace doesn't quite cover it.

Here's what I mean. I grew up in Texas, so naturally (or not so naturally), one of my favorite foods was chicken fried steak. I'm talking about the real Texas chicken fried steak—the kind that's so big that it needs its own plate and is covered in white gravy. (And for the record, if you're going to eat chicken fried steak, use the white gravy, not brown. That's my humble "opinion" as a Texan.) Anyway, I would go to the restaurant, eat a few rolls covered in butter, and order my chicken fried steak with a side of mashed potatoes (also covered in gravy). And I'd throw in some green beans and corn just to make sure I get my veggies. Finally, I'd wash it all down with a big glass of sweet tea—good Southern sweet tea that you could just about stand your spoon up in.

Sounds good, doesn't it? OK, so maybe that doesn't do it for you. I also happen to love Mexican food. And Italian. And Chinese. And Indian. Thai. . . . So whatever your favorite comfort food is, picture that. The question remains the same: What do we do when the server brings it to the table? We pray and thank God for it, which again, we should do.

But we usually ask Him to "bless it to the nourishment of our bodies." To me, that's where we tend to run into trouble. In order for it to nourish our bodies, it has to contain nutrients. But the Standard American Diet (SAD) is calorie dense and nutrient poor.[6] More often than not, we're asking God for a miracle on the level of parting the Red Sea.

Imagine what God is thinking when we ask for him to cause food that is toxic to our bodies to nourish them instead. Some people may argue that as long as you pray over your food, it is sanctified and can't hurt you. But the expanding waistlines and accompanying health problems that plague so many people—including Christ followers—are proof that God isn't honoring that prayer. Is it within God's ability to nourish our bodies with that kind of food? Of course it is. But should we even be asking for that?

The Gospels tell us that Satan tempted Jesus after He had fasted for 40 days. The first temptation was to turn stones into bread. Jesus had to have been starving, but he didn't take the bait. Next, Satan took him to the top of the temple in Jerusalem and challenged Him to jump off so the whole world could see the angels rescue Him (Matthew 4:5-6). Satan actually used a verse from Psalms to make the challenge even more enticing. But again, Jesus didn't fall for it. Instead, he quoted a verse of His own about refusing to put God to the test (Matthew 4:7).

Instead of asking God to defy the laws of nature (like jumping off the top of the temple), perhaps it would be better to ask God to help us choose food that will glorify Him *and* nourish our bodies.

If we agree with Scripture that our body is a temple, that we should never serve other gods, and that we should glorify God in what we eat and drink, it follows that we should be more careful and deliberate about what we put into our bodies. As Nutritionist Heather L. Morgan says, "Every time you eat or drink you are either feeding disease or fighting it."[7] Ask God to help you make wise food choices that bring glory to Him and health to your body. Find someone to hold you accountable to your commitment to a God-honoring nutrition plan.

Food is a gift from God. One that He meant for us to enjoy—according to what He intended for food.

GOD'S FOOD PLAN

In the very first chapter of the Bible, God says, "Behold, I have given you every plant yielding seed that is on the face of all the earth, and every tree with seed in its fruit. You shall have them for food" (Gen 1:29 ESV).

God knew that humans would need food for nourishment. It is a gift from Him. But the original instruction regarding what we should eat was entirely plant-based. Plants provide a great source of vitamins, minerals, proteins, healthy fats, and "phytochemicals," which, by definition, are found only in plants (*phyto* means "plant" in Greek). Phytochemicals contain invaluable and biologically significant substances, such as antioxidants, that many believe reduce the risk of cancer, stroke, metabolic syndrome, and other illnesses. Even today, a healthy diet will consist primarily of natural, unprocessed, unrefined, and often raw plants.

Remember Michael Pollan's advice? "Eat food. Not too much. Mostly plants."

After Noah and his family got off the Ark after The Flood, God allowed meat in our diet for the first time. "Every moving thing that lives shall be food for you. And as I gave you the green plants, I give you everything" (Genesis 9:3 ESV). We don't know exactly why this change occurred, but one common theory is that our environment had changed. Humanity became even more dependent on heavy labor, speed, and physical strength to survive in this new world. As a result, the proteins unique to meat have some benefit.

God also began putting some limits on eating the flesh of animals: "But you shall not eat flesh with its life, that is, its blood" (Genesis 9:4 ESV).

Even though God now allowed the eating of flesh, He created our bodies to run most effectively on a diet consisting mostly, if not entirely, of plants. William C. Roberts, editor in chief of the *American Journal of Cardiology* and medical director of the Baylor University Heart and Vascular Institute, here in the red-blooded state of Texas, says that humans aren't physiologically designed to be meat eaters. Our intestinal length, our need for vitamin C from outside sources, and our ability to sweat link us more closely to herbivores than to carnivorous mammals. "I think the evidence is pretty clear," he says. "If you look at various characteristics of carnivores versus herbivores, it doesn't take a genius to see where humans line up." Our flat (rather than pointed) teeth, the carb-metabolizing enzyme amylase contained in our saliva, and the fact that we, unlike carnivores, can't metabolize uric acid also suggest that we are better adapted to eat plants than animal foods."[8]

God expanded the regulations concerning the consumption of meat in the Mosaic Law. These dietary laws—found in passages like in Leviticus 11 and Deuteronomy 14—distinguished the clean, edible animals from the unclean, inedible animals. I suggest reading those chapters for yourself. The guidelines are pretty extensive, but Dr. Jordan Rubin's book, *The Maker's Diet,* does a great job of this.[9]

In this eye-opening book, Dr. Rubin shares the story of his personal triumph over Crohn's Disease by following God's health rules as lined out in the Old Testament. Clean land animals are ruminants—grazing animals such as cattle, sheep, deer and elk—whose digestive tracts are designed to turn grass that human beings cannot digest into meat that we can. Edible animals had to chew cud and have cloven hooves. Most unclean animals are carnivores or scavengers that can transmit dangerous diseases to human beings. Examples of unclean animals include pigs, rabbits, dogs, cats, horses, and squirrels.

Edible water creatures had to have both fins and scales. This would include species such as salmon, tuna, trout, cod, and mahi mahi. However much of today's most popular seafood—such as shrimp, crab, lobster, catfish, squid, and eels—does not pass that test. Unclean aquatic animals are generally filter feeders. They purify water and concentrate poisonous chemicals, pathologic bacteria, and viruses in their tissues.

Birds that live primarily on insects, grubs, or grains were considered clean, but God said to avoid birds that eat flesh. So, the good list included chicken, turkey, dove, quail, and ducks. Birds on the restricted list were primarily birds of prey, such as falcons, eagles, and owls—along with all scavengers like vultures. (I don't think too many of us are eating them anyway, so not to worry.)

Want to know what insects you can eat? Though not found in most Western diets, insects that have jointed legs above their feet and hop on the ground—such as locusts and grasshoppers—were clean. Does that gross you out? Well, shrimp, crabs, and lobsters are closely related to insects. Technically, they are crustaceans; but they are from the same larger group called arthropods. There is a reason that crawfish are called "mud bugs." They kind of look like bugs, don't they? So, the next time you get a hankering for shrimp, remind yourself that they're basically roaches.

I have a pretty good rule for myself to sum it all up: *If it eats feces, dead things, or its own young, it's off the menu.* You wouldn't want to eat something that had just been munching on a pile of fecal matter, would you?

THE LAW AND GRACE

The Old Testament dietary laws are simultaneously some of the most fascinating and highly disputed pieces of health advice contained in Scripture. You may have heard of them referred to as the "kosher" laws. *Kosher* literally means "fit" or "approved." In orthodox Jewish cultures, the only time you don't need to follow kosher guidelines are situations that save a life. However, if you ask 100 Christians if these guidelines still apply to us today, probably 99 of them will say "no."

I know this because, until a couple of years ago, I would have told you the same thing. My reasoning was the same as most people in the church: As Christians, we are under the New Covenant rather than the Old Covenant. We live by grace, not the law. I would then point to a couple of verses in the New Testament to make my case. I didn't know any Christians still lived by those laws until I dated a girl who was Seventh-Day Adventist. For the 18 months we were together, I gave up unclean meats. Can you imagine going 18 months without real bacon?

Oh, the things we will sacrifice when we're in love.

After we broke up, I went back to my old ways. When I first started writing about biblical health, I didn't bother to dig too deep into the dietary laws—mostly because I didn't want to. In fact, the first time I heard about *The Maker's Diet*, I dismissed it. Eventually, I bought a copy and actually read it. Dr. Rubin began following God's food laws for health reasons and it worked for him. I couldn't very well argue with that.

You may not know this, but Seventh-Day Adventists are renowned for their health.[10] There are little longevity "hot spots" around the world called "Blue Zones." These are areas where people commonly live active lives past the age of 100. There are only five official Blue Zones in the world, and only one of them is in the United States—in Loma Linda, California. Researchers discovered this zone as they were studying a group of Seventh-Day Adventists. They found that the Adventists suffered only a fraction of the diseases and illnesses that plague the rest of the developed world. They also lived much longer and more active lives than the average American.[11]

Loma Linda residents treat their body like a temple and it is paying off for them.[12]

Obviously, they are doing something different. A large part of that "something" turned out to be their commitment to the same dietary laws that allowed many Jewish people to enjoy healthier and longer lives than the surrounding populations for thousands of years.

But in most churches, even suggesting that these 3,000-year-old plus laws could possibly be relevant to 21st-century Christians will quickly get you branded a "legalist"—or worse. I'm ashamed to say I used to say such things, particularly now that I know what it feels like. You see, I've had that label applied to me on more than one occasion by people who haven't even heard me out. I even had a pastor forbid me from even reading Leviticus 11 in his church.

Before looking at what the Mosaic Law says about food and health, we need to clearly understand the function and purpose of the Law in the life of New Testament believers. The first thing we need to understand is that, in Christ, we are free from the Law. This freedom is one of the greatest privileges we have has children of God.

Paul wrote on more than one occasion that the law only served to increase sin and that the "power of sin is the law" (Romans 4:15; 5:13,20; 7:13; 1 Corinthians 15:56). The law reveals our sinfulness, but it does nothing to help us. Quite the contrary, its demand for perfect obedience leaves us condemned and without hope. And that drives us to recognize our need for a Savior. "Therefore the Law has become our tutor to lead us to Christ, so that we may be justified by faith" (Galatians 3:24 NASB). The New Living Translation calls the Law "our guardian" and says it "protected us until we could be made right with God through faith."

But being free from the Law doesn't mean it's not relevant. And it doesn't mean that Christians have no moral imperatives on their life. Paul, who told us we are living under grace (Romans 6:14), immediately said, "What then? Should we sin because we are not under law but under grace? Absolutely not!" (Romans 6:15 HSCB).

We are free from the law, not because it has been done away with, but because Jesus kept it for us perfectly. We have His righteousness. Jesus very plainly said, "Do not think that I have come to abolish the Law or the Prophets; I have not come to abolish them but to fulfill them." (Matt 5:17 ESV)

There is a *big* difference between abolishing something and fulfilling it. The Law still stands because God and His laws are unchanging. "For truly, I say to you, until heaven and earth pass away, not an iota, not a dot, will pass from the Law until all is accomplished." (Matthew 5:18 ESV).

God's Law is still relevant in our live, because it is the system of rules by which God teaches us His will and about how He administers the affairs of the world. It shows us the right way to live, which is exactly what Paul said: "All Scripture is inspired by God and is useful to teach us what is true and to make us realize what is wrong in our lives. It corrects us when we are wrong and teaches us to do what is right" (2 Tim 3:16 NLT)

Unlike the law that revealed and produced sin within us, grace gives us both the desire and the ability to do what is right. "For the grace of God has appeared, bringing salvation for all people, training us to renounce ungodliness and worldly passions, and to live self-controlled, upright, and godly lives in the present age" (Titus 2:11–12 ESV).

What's important for us is to understand God' purpose — His heart — in giving us these rules. What is their purpose? How are they relevant to us today? As it turns out, He gave them to us to improve our health.

Esteemed theologian J. Vernon McGee concluded, "Since God forbade the eating of certain animals and permitted the eating of others, it must be assumed that there was a health factor involved."[13]

The *Expositor's Bible Commentary* said, "It is of much significance to note, in the first place, that a large part of the animals which are forbidden as food are unclean feeders. It is a well-ascertained fact that even the cleanest animal, if its food be unclean, becomes dangerous to health if its flesh be eaten."[14]

Professor Hosmer wrote: "Throughout the entire history of Israel, the wisdom of the ancient lawgivers in these respects has been remarkably shown. In times of pestilence the Jews have suffered far less than others; as regards longevity and general health, they have in every age been noteworthy, and, at the present day, in the life-insurance offices, the life of a Jew is said to be worth much more than that of men of other stock."[15]

The evidence clearly shows that the biblical laws were given for health reasons as well as spiritual, even though Moses and the Israelites wouldn't have understood the health aspect.

THE PURPOSE OF THE DIETARY LAWS

The purpose of the dietary laws is "to make a distinction between the unclean and the clean and between the living creature that may be eaten and the living creature that may not be eaten" (Leviticus 11:47 ESV). This passage beautifully summarizes the dual purpose of Leviticus 11— distinguishing the "clean" from the "unclean" *and* distinguishing the "edible" from the "inedible."

This was not the first time God distinguished between clean and unclean animals. He told Noah to take a pair of every kind of animal onto the ark. But did you know He told Noah to take *seven pairs* of clean animals (Genesis 7:2)? So before God allowed for the eating of meat, there was already a distinction between clean and unclean animals. We are not told how Noah knew the difference between clean and unclean animals, but obviously God communicated it to him in a way he understood.

Some scholars believe the food laws are merely symbolic of the division between Jew and Gentile.[16] But here's where the mistake is made: People often believe this is the only purpose of the dietary laws, so it gets dismissed as irrelevant. This view also seems a bit arbitrary and fails to answer questions about why the divisions were made. McGee countered, "Now it is true that God could have acted in an arbitrary fashion in setting up these lines of separation between clean and unclean, but, ordinarily, God acted for the good of His people. Does history show this to be the case in these matters?"[17] We will see that it does indeed.

Most Christians are familiar with the story of Daniel and his friends, Hananiah, Mishael, and Azariah. You might know them better by their Babylonian names: Shadrach, Meshach, and Abednego. Daniel and his friends decided to obey God's dietary laws rather than fit in with the Babylonian culture and defile themselves (Daniel 1:8). They got permission to eat only vegetables and drink only water for 10 days on the condition that they would then be compared to the other servants who ate from the king's table. After 10 days, Daniel and his friends looked healthier than the other servants and were given permission to continue their diet.

Remember the advice to find out what everyone else is doing and do the opposite? This is a perfect example of how that works out.

What we learn from Daniel 1 is that by following God's guidelines rather than those of the surrounding culture, God blessed Daniel and his friends. In Proverbs 23, Solomon advised: "When you sit down to eat with a ruler, observe carefully what is before you, and put a knife to your throat if you are given to appetite. Do not desire his delicacies, for they are deceptive food" (Proverbs 23:1–3 ESV).

The point? Keep your appetite in check and avoid "deceptive food," even if it means putting a knife to your throat—a reminder perhaps that if you indulge yourself, you are slitting your own throat.[18] I've heard it said that many people dig their own graves with their teeth. History has shown that Israel's dietary laws kept them healthier than their neighbors. In an unpublished book entitled, "The Art of Health" Dr. Peter Rothschild stated:

"It suddenly dawned on us that God, the greatest master nutritionist of all times, has given us an all-purpose diet more than 3000 years ago. . . . There is abundant historic evidence that reveals that the average Israelite, up to the end of the [19th] century, was much longer lived than the average gentile. We wish to emphasize that we are referring to the Israelites up to the end of the last century, because up to those years, the overwhelming majority of Jews obeyed God's laws by and large... it appears that God indeed knew what nourishment to recommend."[19]

During the course of the 20th century, as Jews began to relax their commitments to the health laws, that trend of longevity began to vanish. Conforming to the surrounding cultures removed them from the protection of God's promise: "If you will listen carefully to the voice of the LORD your God and do what is right in his sight, obeying his commands and keeping all his decrees, then I will not make you suffer any of the diseases I sent on the Egyptians; for I am the LORD who heals you." (Exodus 15:26 NLT)

As long as God's people followed His rules, He protected them. They were able to avoid the diseases God placed on other people. In a *New York Medical Journal* published in 1901, there is an article entitled "The Comparative Pathology of the Jews" by Dr. Maurice Fishberg. Fishberg noted, "On carefully considering the above facts and figures, we are forced to agree with W. L. Ripley, that the Jews show an 'unprecedented tenacity of life.'" [20] Dr. Fishberg went on to demonstrate "that the Jews are relatively less likely to be attacked by disease. When we turn again to the causes of death among the Jews, we find that the most dangerous diseases, as tuberculosis, pneumonia, nephritis, typhoid, malaria, etc. (except diabetes), claim a proportionately smaller number of victims from among the Jews than from among non-Jews."[21]

When they started giving in to their surrounding culture and relaxing on His principles, they began to pay the price. It turns out God gave us His dietary laws not just as a mere symbolic separation of His people, but to actually improve our health—a fact that we will see has now been proven by modern science.

AHEAD OF THEIR TIME

Modern science is finally catching up to what God said in His Word thousands of years ago. When the latest scientific discoveries point to intelligent design in the universe and force atheists and agnostics to acknowledge the existence of a Creator, we applaud. Dr. Robert Jastrow, founder of NASA's Institute for Space Studies—and an agnostic—acknowledged: "For the scientist who has lived by his faith in the power of reason, the story ends like a bad dream. He has scaled the mountains of ignorance; he is about to conquer the highest peak; as he pulls himself over the final rock, he is greeted by a band of theologians who have been sitting there for centuries."[22]

If agnostics like Dr. Jastrow can admit when the evidence contradicts their pre-conceived bias, why is it so difficult for Christians, who should be more concerned with truth than anyone?

Modern scientific studies have presented convincing evidence that there are serious health risks associated with eating animals God tells us are unclean and inedible. It has been proven that most of these animals carry parasites and disease. In answer to his question of whether or not God acted for the good of His people when giving us the food laws, J. Vernon McGee began by saying, "Well, the interesting thing we will find is that the animals which were forbidden to be eaten were largely unclean feeders. The animals rejected by the Mosaic system are more liable to disease."[23]

Dr. Kellogg pointed out: "One of the greatest discoveries of modern science is the fact that a large number of diseases to which animals are liable are due to the presence of low forms of parasitic life. To such diseases those which are unclean in their feeding will be especially exposed, while none will perhaps be found wholly exempt. Another discovery of recent times which has a no less important bearing on the question raised by this chapter is the now ascertained fact that many of these parasitic diseases are common to both animals and men, and may be communicated from the former to the latter."[24]

Both Dr. McGee and Dr. Kellogg quoted Dr. Noel de Mussy in a statement presented to the Paris Academy of Medicine: "The idea of parasitic and infectious maladies, which has conquered so great a position in modern pathology, appears to have greatly occupied the mind of Moses and to have dominated all his hygienic rules. He excluded from Hebrew dietary animals particularly liable to parasites; and as it is in the blood that the germs and spores of infectious disease circulate, he orders that they must be drained of their blood before serving for food."[25,26]

We also know that the flesh of unclean animals is highly toxic. In 1953, David Macht, M.D., an experimental biologist at Johns Hopkins University whose methods of assessing pharmacological toxicity are still used today, published research findings from a study he entitled, "An

Experimental Pharmacological Appreciation of Leviticus XI and Deuteronomy XIV."[27]

Dr. Macht wrote, "In studying muscle extracts of fresh meats from various species of animals some very interesting findings were made."[28] Interesting indeed. Dr. Macht tested the flesh of 54 kinds of fish, 21 animals, and 14 birds. What was "interesting" is that every single animal God said was unclean tested out as toxic, while every single animal that God said was clean tested out as non-toxic. Dr. Macht's tests confirmed the biblical position that those animals, birds, and fish listed as "unclean" were not healthy for human consumption. There was a 100 percent correlation between Israel's dietary laws and the scientific study!

His conclusion? "Every word in the Hebrew Scriptures is well chosen and carries valuable knowledge and deep significance."[29] So, it turns out that God was right. Why should that surprise us?

Yes, the New Testament teaches that we are no longer judged regarding what foods we eat (Colossians 2:16), but nutrition science continues to confirm that God's rules make for the healthiest diet.

We all know the saying, "You are what you eat." Taken a step further, you are also what your food eats. Most animals listed as inedible are scavengers. Obviously, an animal that eats filth won't have very healthy flesh. Pigs, for example, will eat almost anything they can find, including their own young and sick or dead pigs from the same pen. That's not just nasty; it's also dangerous. And remember my rule about anything that eats feces or its own young being off the menu? Is it starting to make a little more sense?

Even if the Bible were silent on this subject, there is more than enough scientific evidence to motivate a prudent person toward avoiding, or at least limiting the "unclean" animals for health reasons.

THE LAWS WE DON'T QUESTION

As many objections as I've had about teaching the dietary laws, I've never once had someone object to teaching the hygiene and sanitation laws. As with the laws regarding food, the sanitation laws were thousands of years ahead of their time! The medical instructions given by Moses to the Israelites some 3,500 years ago were not only far superior to the practices of contemporary cultures, but they also exceeded medical standards practiced as recently as 100 years ago. Until recently there was no way for these laws to be fully understood until the invention of the microscope, which led to the discovery of bacteria and other microscopic pathogens.

So, where did Moses get this advanced information? From God, of course.

For centuries doctors denied the possibility of unseen disease-carrying particles. That changed in the mid-19th century when Louis Pasteur proved that diseases were carried by microorganisms that were foreign to the body. This new understanding of germs and bacteria led to improved sanitation practices that resulted in a dramatic decrease in the mortality rate. Yet, under God's instructions, the Jewish people had been practicing them for thousands of years. Immediately after he gave the dietary laws, God began giving us laws concerning cleanliness (Leviticus 12–15).

People who touched a dead or diseased person or animal were commanded to wash themselves and their clothes—even if they only touched the garments or secretions from a sick person. They also had to avoid contact with others. Any clothes that were contaminated had to be washed or burned. Buildings that showed signs of mold or that had housed sick individuals were cleaned and repaired to prevent the spread of disease. Sometimes, the buildings even had to be destroyed.

Any porous vessels that came into contact with dead animals were also destroyed, since they would be contaminated with bacteria the Israelites didn't even know existed. They also practiced quarantine to prevent the spread of diseases such as leprosy. People showing signs of sickness had to be isolated and were not allowed back into society until they were examined by a priest and declared well.

These are all important principles of sanitation and cleanliness that are still practiced today.

In Deuteronomy 23:9–14, we learn that human wastes were to be buried away from human dwellings. We don't really think about that in our world of indoor plumbing, but try to imagine life without it. Our grandparents and great-grandparents, even some of our parents, are old enough to remember outhouses. The benefits of sanitary waste disposal are widely understood, but there are still parts of the world, especially in poverty-stricken areas, where it's not practiced. History is filled with epidemics of typhus, cholera, dysentery, and other diseases that are linked to the improper disposal of human waste. We know this now, but God provided these instructions thousands of years before we knew why.

These laws also preserved the Jewish people through the horrendously dark period of the Black Plague that killed approximately 40-60 percent of the population of Europe. Jews reportedly died at only half the rate of Christians.[30] That's because the Mosaic Law imposed a sanitary standard on Jews that went far beyond the ordinary sanitary standard of most medieval Europeans. "For instance, Jewish law compels one to wash his or her hands many times throughout the day. In the general medieval world, a person could go half his or her life without ever washing his hands. According to Jewish law, one could not eat food without washing one's hands, leaving the bathroom and after any sort of intimate human contact. At least once a week, a Jew bathed for the Sabbath. Furthermore, Jewish law prevents the Jew from reciting blessings and saying prayers by an open pit at latrines and at places with a foul odor. The sanitary conditions in the Jewish neighborhood, primitive as it may be by today's standards, was always far superior to the general sanitary conditions."[31]

Dr. Fishberg observed, "This peculiar resistance of the Jews to the noxious effects of contagious disease has been noted already in the middle ages, especially during the great epidemics in Europe of the plague known as the 'Black Death.' At that time, they suffered severely, because of the fact that they were affected by the pestilence to a less degree and had a proportionately smaller mortality than the Christians. The Jews were accused of being the special emissaries of Satan in causing the plague; it was said that their immunity was due to a special protection by Satan."[32]

In addition to the low mortality rate of the Jews during the plague, Dr. Kellogg brought out, "In our own day, in the recent cholera epidemic in Italy, a correspondent of the Jewish Chronicle testifies that the Jews enjoyed almost absolute immunity, at least from fatal attack."[33] God's wisdom given through Moses for the prevention of infectious disease prompted Dr. John Scudder to exclaim, "What an extraordinary prescience is this! ... The Mosaic law in reality anticipated modern science by several thousand years. Its inscribed precepts included laws established for the prevention of [disease]."[34]

LEGALISTIC OR LIFE GIVING?

So, is it really legalistic to follow the Mosaic Law for health reasons? That depends on your motivation. You see, obeying the Mosaic Law doesn't make you a legalist; obeying it with the wrong motivation does.

Legalism could be defined as any attempt to rely on self-effort to either attain or maintain our justification before God. In Paul's Epistle to the Galatians, he warned them sternly about such false understandings of the gospel: "How foolish can you be? After starting your new lives in the Spirit, why are you now trying to become perfect by your own human effort?" (Galatians 3:3 NLT). Legalism always seems to have one primary characteristic: It's theology denies that Christ is sufficient for salvation, believing that some additional element of self-effort, merit, or faithfulness on our part is necessary. Therefore, any teaching that says "faith plus anything else" is legalism.

As stated earlier, there is no question that Christ's death eliminated the ceremonial significance of the dietary laws. But Christ's sacrifice in no way changed the anatomy of a human being or the design and habits of unclean animals. Unclean animals were unhealthy to eat in the days of Moses and are just as unhealthy for us today.

ALL FOODS CLEAN?

This is where the argument comes in that Jesus declared all foods clean: "And he said to them, 'Then are you also without understanding? Do you not see that whatever goes into a person from outside cannot defile him, since it enters not his heart but his stomach, and is expelled?' (Thus he declared all foods clean)" (Mark 7:18–19 ESV).

But is that what Jesus was really saying, that the animals God had previously declared unclean are now clean? Was Jesus correcting an error on the part of His Father? Of course not. When you compare Mark 7 to Matthew 15, you see that Jesus was not even addressing the question of clean and unclean animals. The issue was eating without washing the hands.

In Matthew 15:2, Jesus was dealing with a controversy by the Pharisees, who insisted that the disciples ceremonially wash their hands before they ate food. This is a hygiene issue, not a food issue. Christ condemned their hypocritical tradition in verses 3-10, declaring that the Pharisees worshipped God in vain by emphasizing manmade laws—the "tradition of the elders"—as His law. Jesus drew a clear distinction between the Old Testament, which was the commandment of God, and the tradition of the Pharisees, which consisted of merely human "add-ons."

From there, in verse 11, He made the statement about defilement coming out of man, not going in.

Peter then asked Jesus to explain this parable. Notice how Jesus expounded on this: "And he said, 'Are you also still without understanding? Do you not see that whatever goes into the mouth passes into the stomach and is expelled? But what comes out of the mouth proceeds from the heart, and this defiles a person. For out of the heart come evil thoughts, murder, adultery, sexual immorality, theft, false witness, slander. These are what defile a person. But to eat with unwashed hands does not defile anyone'" (Matt 15:16–20 ESV).

Now we begin to understand the situation. Jesus knew that the Pharisees had murderous thoughts in their hearts against him and that they were more concerned with making Him look bad than fixing their own evil hearts. Jesus called out their sins by name and declared that those were the things that defiled a man—not eating with unwashed hands. A few chapters later, Jesus chastised the Pharisees again for their hypocrisy and blindness. They were focused on the wrong things. They appeared to be clean, but inside they were full of all kinds of nastiness (Matthew 23:23–28).

Notice what Jesus says—and what He does not say. He says they were wrong in their focus, not in what they were doing. The Pharisees asked why the disciples didn't wash their hands before eating. By itself, it's actually a legitimate question; but that wasn't their focus—and that's what got them into trouble.

Let me ask you a question: Do you think it's a good idea to wash your hands before you eat? How about this, let's say you go out to eat at a restaurant and you notice someone in the bathroom who doesn't wash their hands before they leave. Is that gross? What if it turns out that person is your server? Would you want them serving your food? That's a health code violation for a reason.

The disciples should have washed their hands—not because it was the law or defiled them, but because it presented health risks.

PETER'S VISION

Perhaps the most common passage of Scripture used to prove that Jesus abolished the dietary laws is found in Acts 10 and 11. Peter received a vision of a sheet coming down from heaven containing unclean animals. Three times, he was told to kill and eat. But Peter, who was one of Jesus' inner circle along with James and John, understood that this was wrong and resisted! Each time, Peter objected that he had never eaten anything unclean. Each time God replied, "What God has made clean, do not call common." Finally, the sheet was taken back up into heaven.

To understand the context of this passage, we need to make some critical observations. First, Peter's resistance to eating unclean animals demonstrated that during his entire three and a half years with Jesus, he had never seen or heard anything that led him to accept unclean meats. In other words, Jesus had not changed the prohibition against eating the forbidden animals. If He had, Peter would have known about it and would not have responded as he did. So, Jesus' statement in Mark 7 did not abolish the Old Testament law. Jesus and the disciples continued to follow the dietary restrictions.

Second, the context of Acts 10 reveals that Peter himself wasn't sure what the vision meant. Verse 17 tells us that Peter "was inwardly perplexed as to what the vision that he had seen might mean" (ESV). While Peter was pondering the meaning of the vision, three Gentiles who had been sent by Cornelius arrived at his home. Peter was prompted by the Spirit to go with them. The next day, Peter returned with them to Caesarea, where Cornelius had his family and friends gathered to welcome the apostle.

On meeting Cornelius and hearing his story, Peter finally understood the meaning of his vision. It's important to see that Peter's own interpretation of the vision was not that it was okay for Christians to eat pigs, shellfish, and other unclean animals. Instead, his interpretation in Acts 10:28 was, "God has shown me that I should not call any *person* common or unclean" (ESV, emphasis added). The result was that the Church started preaching the Gospel to the Gentiles, who were symbolized by the unclean animals.

God used the vision of the sheet to teach Peter that salvation was available to the Gentiles, not just the Jews. So, the sheet and the animals had nothing to do with eating and drinking. The vision was addressing evangelism, not food.

What a dramatic lesson for that early church! And it's a lesson that all of us should learn. From this moment on, be quick to correct those who try to apply this vision to any cleansing of unclean animals. It actually proves the opposite—and then presses home one of the greatest lessons for Christians everywhere–every individual has equal worth before God, so we need to make every effort to win every person to Christ.

RECEIVED WITH THANKSGIVING

> "For everything created by God is good, and nothing is to be rejected if it is received with thanksgiving, for it is made holy by the word of God and prayer." (1 Timothy 4:4–5 ESV)

You may then bring up Paul's words to Timothy here and argue that as long as we receive food with thanksgiving and ask God to bless it, it's all good. First, let's consider again the context by backing up a couple of verses.

"Now the Spirit expressly says that in later times some will depart from the faith by devoting themselves to deceitful spirits and teachings of demons, through the insincerity of liars whose consciences are seared, who forbid marriage and require abstinence from foods that God created to be received with thanksgiving by those who believe and know the truth. For everything created by God is good, and nothing is to be rejected if it is received with thanksgiving, for it is made holy by the word of God and prayer." (1 Timothy 4:1–5 ESV)

In 1 Timothy 3, Paul had been talking about qualifications for elders and deacons, as well as how believers should behave in the household of God. He then went on to talk about training for godliness and even mentioned that bodily training (exercise) has a certain degree of value. So, did he follow that up by saying that teaching about food and health is a doctrine of demons? On the contrary, the goal of the enemy is to steal, kill, and destroy. The enemy doesn't want you healthy; the enemy wants you sick, incapacitated and dead.

And did you catch that qualifier in there — "foods that God created to be received with thanksgiving." The foods that God created would include the things that God meant to be food. Unclean animals were never meant to be food for God's people. But if someone tells you God forbids the eating of broccoli, that would be a doctrine of demons.

For those of you who are parents of small children, let me ask you to imagine something with me: Let's pretend your child wakes up tomorrow morning and decides to fix their own breakfast. But when you walk into the kitchen, you discover that they have filled an extra-large bowl with frosted cocoa sugar bombs with lots of extra sugar on top. And for good measure, they threw on a couple of scoops of ice cream and some hot fudge. And since we all know that sweet and salty go together so well, they added a pile of bacon.

Now, how would you react? And what would you say when they told you it was okay because they were going to ask God to bless it?

You'd *never* let them get away with that! But to a certain degree, that's exactly how many of us act when it comes to our favorite foods. We think it's fine, as long as we ask God to bless it. But I think you'll have a hard time backing that up from what Paul wrote to Timothy—or anything else in Scripture.

PROPER PERSPECTIVE

I know some of this probably hits close to home. But it's important to understand that when it comes to our health—especially our food choices—we are driven by forces deep below the surface: "The purpose in a man's heart is like deep water" (Proverbs 20:5 ESV).

The problem is that we are "looking for love in all the wrong places" to quote a famous song. In his book, *Food and Love*, Christian relationship expert Gary Smalley, highlights the cycle that many of us live in where the health of our diet and the health of our relationships contribute to one another. We try to fill a void in our hearts with food.[35] That is why you often hear people talk about being emotional eaters. Understanding why we do what we do can help us in fixing what we do.

I remember as a high school student asking my youth minister how far was "too far" when it came to relationships with the opposite sex. His answer humbled me and showed me the error of my thinking. He said, "You're asking the wrong question. Instead of asking how far you can stretch God's law without breaking it, you should be asking how can I best glorify God in my relationships." Ouch. That hurt—not because it was mean or legalistic, but because I knew in my heart that he was right.

The same is true when it comes to food. Remember the verse, "So, whether you eat or drink, or whatever you do, do all to the glory of God" (1 Corinthians 10:31 ESV)? The question really isn't, "Can I eat this?" Instead, it's "Should I eat this?" Again, Paul reminds us, "You say, 'I am allowed to do anything'—but not everything is good for you. And even though 'I am allowed to do anything,' I must not become a slave to anything" (1 Corinthians 6:12 NLT). The immediate context of this verse is sexual, but it is a general principle for all of our physical drives.

The question here is one of authority and power: Who's in control, you or your appetites? Are you a slave to your desires or to God? Is this something that is good for you, or something that will harm you? Like any good parent, God only establishes rules for our benefit. He gives us guidelines because He loves us and wants the best for us. In their proper context, no New Testament passage forbids following the dietary laws for health reasons, and those health reasons are as valid today as they were 3,500 years ago.

If you think about God's food laws as restrictions that require an unbearable sacrifice, you're going to struggle. But what if you turn it around? Focus on all the amazing and delicious foods God *did* give you— how much better you will feel when you stick to them. The bottom line is that in order to live well, we must change our habits. We must redefine our approach to food. We can't simply do whatever we feel like doing because our bodies belong to God, not to us.

God is the author of the biblical health laws. The Bible reveals that God does not change (Malachi 3:6), which means that His fundamental laws do not change. The laws of biology did not suddenly change, or stop operating, when Jesus came on the scene. The same factors that caused or prevented disease in the days of Moses still operate today.

To be our best, we must suppress the desire for what feels good in the moment and pursue what best allows us to serve our Creator. We live for a higher purpose and calling. Fortunately, God has given us an instruction book, The Bible, that tells us where the boundaries are. If we ignore His guidelines, we will pay the price in our bodies and in our lives, but if we live our lives according to His guidelines, He will satisfy our desires and give us abundant life. We will be fit and healthy, live longer, enjoy a higher quality of life, increased energy and improved mood. We will be fully alive!

CHAPTER 8

FOODOLOGY

Let food be your medicine and medicine be your food.[1]
— HIPPOCRATES, The Founder of Modern Medicine

The doctor of the future will no longer treat the human frame with drugs, but rather will cure and prevent disease with nutrition.[2]
— THOMAS EDISON

There seems to be a lot of confusion around nutrition—a subject that God intended to be very simple. There are plenty of books and theories out there so it's hard to know what to do, especially when so many of them offer conflicting advice. Should your diet be low-fat or low-carb? Should you follow a Paleo Diet, Vegan Diet, Macrobiotic Diet, or Ketogenic Diet? What about regional diets like the Mediterranean Diet and the Brazilian Diet? And what should we do about counting calories?

It's confusing, I know. When you add in all of the advertising and "studies" thrown at you by the food industry—including many that are designed to mislead you—it's that much more perplexing.

So, what diet should you follow? How about a plan designed specifically for your body by the One who created it and loves you? It works regardless of your body type or blood type, whether you are skinny or overweight. It will heal your body and give you more strength and energy and endurance. It will improve your mood. It will normalize your blood sugar and cholesterol all by itself. It virtually eliminates the risk of heart disease, diabetes, and cancer—and if you already have these conditions, it is remarkably effective at reversing them.

This plan will boost your immune system so that when everyone around you is catching colds or the flu, your body will be able to fight it off—like it was designed to do. And on those rare occasions when you do get sick, your recovery will be exponentially faster. Want to know what it is? Michael Pollan already summarized it for us nicely—*"Eat food. Not too much. Mostly plants."*

I told you, God intended for it to be simple. Eat food, meaning *real* food. Food that is whole and natural. Food that once was alive and, therefore, has life in it. Food that your great-grandparents would recognize as food.

Not too much. That one's pretty self-explanatory. Don't overeat. Don't be a glutton. But don't worry—you're much less likely to overeat when you're eating real food. It's the processed foods that were engineered to trick your body into overeating that are the problem. For example, have you ever seen anyone binge on apples or carrots or kale? Probably not.

Mostly plants. Again, self-explanatory. When God created Adam and Eve, the food He gave them to eat consisted entirely of plants. That's the original design of our bodies. So even though God extended our diets beyond plants, we still tend to perform better with a primarily plant-based diet.

What about all of those other diets? Do they work? Sure—for some people, some of the time. The problem with picking one diet system and then saying that everyone should eat that way is that we are not all the same. What works for me may not work for you and vice-versa. *Bio-individuality* is a term coined by Joshua Rosenthal, founder of the Institute for Integrative Nutrition, where I am in school. It recognizes that there is no one-size-fits-all way of eating. There are a number of factors that determine what is best for you, and it will very likely change in different seasons of your life. General guidelines exist, but individuals have freedom within those guidelines.

When I work with clients, I have them fill out a little questionnaire. Then, I talk through it with them to help them figure out the best workout and diet program to reach their goals. As I mentioned earlier, when I work with people who list weight-loss as their primary goal, I always ask, "Do you just want to lose weight, or do you want to experience overall health?" That question is usually met with a puzzled, "What's the difference?" look. It's actually a huge difference. Most people equate weight-loss with improved health, but that's not necessarily the case. Weight is only one indicator of health, and it's not even the best one. There are lots of things you can do to lose weight and not all of them are healthy, in fact, some of them are downright dangerous. Remember Fen-Phen?

My approach has always been to focus on overall health. When you work on the things that improve your health—faith, food, fitness, focus, and fellowship—you tend to end up with the physique you're supposed to have. Weight-loss is a byproduct of doing the right things.

Nutrition is pretty amazing! The more I learn about nutrition and how the body uses food to maintain and repair itself, the more it causes me to marvel and worship our Creator. You know the saying, "You are what you eat?" It's absolutely true. I remember Christian comedian Mike Warnke saying, "If you eat a lot of fat, greasy food, you'll end up a fat, greasy dude." I thought that was hilarious; and at the time, I was a fat, greasy dude. (Well, maybe not greasy.)

But think about it . . . what you eat helps define who you become. Everything—your skin, your muscles, your bones, your internal organs, your nerves, every cell in your body—is created from what you eat and drink. Everything. There's nothing else to build with. Even when you were a baby in your mother's womb, you were created cell by cell by everything your mother ate and drank. That's why pre-natal nutrition is so important. Plus, what you eat and drink also creates the building blocks for every chemical in your body, including the ones that regulate mood, mental clarity, and focus.

Take a good look in the mirror. Do you like what you see? How's your skin? Your hair—unless you're like me and you don't have any? How clear are your eyes? Do you look and feel inflamed—swelling, redness, itching, pain? Think about how you feel. How are your energy levels? What sort of mood have you been in? All of these things and more are determined by what you give your body as building blocks.

So, what fuel have you been using? What have you eaten for the past week? Was it pizza and sodas for dinner, or a giant bacon double cheeseburger for lunch, or donuts and coffee on the way to work? Did it come out of a box or can? Are those things you really believe your body can use to build the best version of you?

Now, let's talk about that bowl of fresh organic fruit you had for breakfast. Or the big, fresh, leafy green salad loaded with fresh raw veggies and seeds and nuts with the delicious homemade salad dressing drizzled on top. Or how about the dinner of grilled wild-caught salmon with steamed broccoli or roasted asparagus and quinoa? Imagine how much better your body would look and feel with fuel like that.

What did you drink? Did you drink a lot of heavily sweetened chemical concoctions? And, no, diet drinks aren't better. They're actually much worse. I'll get to that in a bit. Imagine what a vat of chemical poisons does to your body. What if, instead you drank lots of fresh, pure filtered water every day?

Remember the story of the Three Little Pigs? Did you build your house with straw and hay or did you build it with bricks? Whatever your choices, ask yourself these questions: *Is this what I want to be built from? Is this who*

I want to be? Am I building a body that is less prone to illness and injury or more prone? The bottom line is this: "Every time you eat or drink you are either feeding disease or fighting it."[3] If you truly want to maximize your health, you've really got zero wiggle room. Every single choice is either a good one or a bad one. There is no middle ground.

So, if you want to be fully alive, here are the rules again: *Eat food. Not too much. Mostly plants.* Or in the words of Darin Olien, author of *SuperLife: The 5 Forces That Will Make You Healthy, Fit, and Eternally Awesome,* "Eat a wide variety of whole, fresh, clean foods—mostly vegetables, fruits, beans, nuts, seeds, grains, sprouts, and healthy fats. Eat a lot of it raw."[4]

LIFE OR DEATH

Life or death, health or disease, it's your choice. Seriously. You get to choose. Let's just start with the number one killer in America—heart disease. According to the CDC, heart disease kills more than 600,000 Americans every year. In 2014, the number was 614,348.[5]

Dr. Caldwell Esselstyn Jr., former director of the cardiovascular prevention and reversal program at The Cleveland Clinic Wellness Institute, and one of the world's foremost authorities on cardiovascular health describes heart disease as a "completely preventable foodborne illness." He says you can become "heart attack proof"—regardless of your family history.[6] In a one-hour documentary, "Dr. Sanjay Gupta Reports: The Last Heart Attack," Dr. Esselstyn tells Dr. Gupta, "It's a foodborne illness, and we're never going to end the epidemic with stents, with bypasses, with the drugs, because none of it is treating causation of the illness."[7]

Dr. Esselstyn strongly advises against waiting to change your diet until after you develop symptoms of heart disease because most heart attacks strike with little or no warning. He says, "The reason you don't wait until you have heart disease to eat this way is often, sadly, the first symptom of your heart disease may be your sudden death."[8]

That's what my doctor told me after my dramatic transformation—that I had not only saved my life, I had probably given myself decades more of good life.

Cancer runs a very close second to heart disease in the number of lives it claims every year and is regarded by many as the most dreaded of all diseases. It's also highly preventable. According to the CDC, the number of cancer-related deaths in 2014 was 591,699.[9] It's estimated that diet causes about one-third of all cancer cases. Just to put it into perspective, that's almost as many as tobacco. And that's not counting the cancers that could have been *prevented* by proper diet, just the ones *caused* by poor diet. Yes, there is a difference. There is a strong link between cancer and chronic inflammation in the body. The good news is that God has provided us with a whole host of cancer-fighting, anti-inflammatory chemical compounds in nature—and He put them in food.

So, if we take the roughly 1.2 million deaths from heart disease and cancer, add to it the 133,000 from strokes; the 147,000 from chronic lower respiratory disease; and 77,000 from diabetes, we're left with the cold, hard fact that more than 1.5 million Americans die every year because they made the wrong choices. The vast majority of those diseases could have been prevented or treated through proper diet and exercise, so we are literally digging our own graves with our teeth.

THE HEALING POWER OF FOOD

While the wisdom of Hippocrates, the founder of modern medicine, stated that food should be our medicine, most doctors know very little about nutrition. On average, medical schools provide about 19 hours of nutrition education. Nineteen hours. That's it. So, unless they have done their own research, most doctors simply won't know. Sadly, they are so overworked and stressed that they don't have time to do the research. That's beginning to change and those who are doing the research are discovering that Hippocrates was right—food is medicine.

Unlike anything else, food has the power to heal us. It is the most potent and effective medicine available with the power to prevent and heal most of the chronic illnesses that plague our society. The link between our food and our health is absolute, and its effect is so immediate and so profound that you would think we would be more aware of what is going on in our own bodies. Yet most of us are completely clueless. We have no idea that our food choices are responsible for our health or our lack thereof. If you want to feel better, have more energy, be less prone to illness and disease, even reverse certain diseases, it's time to understand that all of these conditions are fueled by what we put in our bodies.

Do we really doubt that a cheeseburger and a vibrant green salad have different effects on our body? Food is more than just calories. Food instructs us. Have you ever heard someone say that they have "fat genes" or that they are genetically predisposed to certain diseases? That may be true to a certain point, but what we eat has more to do with it than our genes. In fact, even if you had all 32 genes associated with obesity (highly unlikely), it would still only add about 22 pounds to your weight. At best, these genes account for only 9 percent of obesity cases.

Of all of the factors that lead to obesity, the least influential is genetics.[10] That's because our food determines how our genes express themselves. There is a whole new science called *nutrigenomics* that studies how food affects our genes. Think of our cells as little microscopic cities. A lot is going on at the cellular level, and the molecules in your food provide instructions that tell every cell what to do at every moment. Less than 5 percent of chronic illness and disease is related to your genes. That means that more than 95 percent is due to what your genes are exposed to over your lifetime. That's called your "exposome."[11]

The exposome refers to the sum total of environmental exposures from the time you were conceived onward. That includes everything you eat, drink, breathe, think, and feel—and all of the toxins you are exposed to in our environment. Then you have your microbiome—the 2 to 6 pounds of essential bacteria that live in the human body. "An ever-growing number of studies have demonstrated that changes in the composition of our microbiomes correlate with numerous disease states, raising the possibility that manipulation of these communities could be used to treat disease."[12] What this means is that even though we have genetic predispositions, each of us has nearly complete control over our health. How healthy we are depends, for the most part, on what we put into our mouths.

That's good news. That's something we can control.

For example, if we want to prevent cancer, we can eat foods that contain cancer-fighting chemicals. Foods like tomatoes, grapefruit, watermelon and guava contain a micronutrient family called carotenoids. Carotenoids are plant pigments responsible for bright red, yellow, and orange hues in many fruits and vegetables, but they have numerous health benefits. The most common carotenoids in North American diets are α-carotene, β-carotene, β-cryptoxanthin, lutein, zeaxanthin, and lycopene. Carotenoids, and lycopene in particular, have been shown to help keep the liver, prostate, breast, colon, and lungs healthy.[13]

Grapes, berries, and peanuts contain a chemical called resveratrol. Resveratrol is a powerful antioxidant that has been shown to reduce inflammation in the body. It also helps protect your cells from free radical damage. Free radicals are unstable molecules produced in the body as byproducts of cellular reactions, metabolism of foods, breathing and other vital functions.[14] Free radicals ultimately harm and age the body over time because they damage (oxidize) DNA, cellular membranes, lipids (fats) stored within blood vessels and enzymes.[15]

Resveratrol also helps lower blood pressure, and inhibit the spread of cancer, especially prostate cancer. It is also unique among antioxidants because it has the ability to cross the blood-brain barrier. The blood brain barrier is a highly selective semipermeable membrane barrier that separates the circulating blood from the brain extracellular fluid in the central nervous system (CNS).[16] Think of it as a security system for your brain. Because resveratrol has the ability to cross this barrier it is uniquely able to repair and protect your brain and central nervous system. It has also been shown to help prevent Alzheimer's disease.[17]

Red grapes, citrus fruits, berries, broccoli, and leafy green vegetables all contain quercitin. It's also found in tea and wine. Quercitin is considered to be one of the most abundant antioxidants in the human diet and plays a vital role in fighting free radical damage, the effects of aging, and inflammation.

Cruciferous vegetables, such as broccoli, kale and Brussels sprouts, provide us with sulforaphane. This one is actually really cool because it's a compound not actually contained in the plant. It is produced when the enzyme myrosinase (found in saliva) transforms glucoraphanin—a glucosinolate—into sulforaphane when the plant is chewed. That allows the two compounds to mix and react.[18] That's a lot of words, I know, and it's easy to get lost in them, but bear with me. I know my eyes went crossed the first time I read them. The important thing to remember is there is stuff in our saliva that mixes with stuff in the broccoli and they combine to make something completely new—that something is called sulforaphane.

And that's just the beginning. As Darin Olien explains:

> The sulforaphane then activates two hundred different genes, some of them protecting us from cancer and others preventing the disease's spread. Sulforaphane has been found to hinder the growth of breast cancer and prostate cancer cells specifically, although its benefits appear to extend to genes everywhere in the body. It kills cancer stem cells. It normalizes DNA methylation, a process that regulates gene expression. It kills an enzyme that damages cartilage.[19]

When I first learned about this, I marveled at the awesome genius of our amazing God. We get a powerful, healing, cancer-fighting chemical compound from broccoli—even though it isn't actually in broccoli, but is created and released when we chew broccoli. Talk about mind-blowing!

Of course, the catch is you have to actually eat broccoli.

As with all of these amazing compounds, you need to get them from food sources for them to be effective. Synthetic versions just aren't the same. Your body knows what a blueberry is, but it's not so sure about a man-made chemical. Besides, you really can't improve on God's plan. His plan is for us to eat real food, meaning the kinds of food he intended for us to eat.

So, what are real foods? Basically anything that is whole, fresh, clean, and unprocessed. Anything else is fake food—deceptive food. Solomon, the wisest man to ever live, warned us to be mindful of what we eat and who is offering it to us. "When you sit down to eat with a ruler, observe carefully what is before you, and put a knife to your throat if you are given to appetite. Do not desire his delicacies, for they are deceptive food" (Proverbs 23:1–3 ESV). These verses remind us to be discerning in how we deal with others and not allow them to influence us by the extravagance of the food they offer, but they also speak to us about controlling our appetites. And as one writer observed, "we live in an affluent society that has the "king's food" available to the average person. Doctors are now attributing many of our modern-day ailments to the Western diet of too many fats, sweets, and junk food. Instead of eating our foods in their natural forms, as God created them, they are highly processed with a multitude of unhealthy additives. We are a nation addicted to sweet, salty, greasy and rich foods. These would qualify as deceitful foods."[20]

Deceptive food is destructive. It robs us of health and energy and vitality. Real food nourishes. Real food heals.

CARB CONFUSION

Carbohydrates have gotten a pretty bad rap over the last 20 years or so, and the low-carb craze has created a lot of confusion. While eating too many of the wrong kind of carbs can lead to weight gain and other health problems, carbohydrates are essential to a proper diet. Carbohydrates are the body's main source of energy as they are broken down into glucose in the digestive tract. Glucose is the sole source of energy for the brain under normal conditions and is essential in maintaining healthy nerve tissue.

All plant foods contain carbohydrates, but you need to make sure you are getting the right kinds. Those primarily come from fruits and vegetables. Whole grains, beans, and lentils are also good carbs, but they're also starchy, so you've got to eat them in moderation. On the other hand, you can and should load up on non-starchy vegetables. In fact, they should make up at least half of your diet.

Plant foods do more than anything else to improve your health. They are the primary source of vitamins and minerals. They are also our only source of phytonutrients, which are extremely potent chemicals that fight inflammation, detoxify our systems, and balance our blood sugar. Fruit is another excellent source of phytonutrients, and the darker and richer the colors of the fruit the better. Lower-glycemic fruits such as cherries, grapefruit, apples, and berries are best.

Good sources of complex carbohydrates include: leafy green vegetables, fresh fruit, sweet potatoes, legumes, quinoa, and brown rice. If you want bread, try a sprouted grain bread like the Ezekiel 4:9 brand. You'll find it in the frozen bread section of your grocery store. Or you can buy an heirloom grain, like einkorn wheat, and make your own bread. These are better for you.

The problem is that most Americans get the majority of their carbs from eight sources: unhealthy drinks (like soft drinks), pastries, pizza, snack chips, white rice, white breads, beer, and frozen potatoes (like French fries). Not exactly a recipe for health. These high-carbohydrate foods are low in vitamins, minerals, and fiber. Plus, they may ultimately lead to insulin resistance and diabetes. Even if the body doesn't develop insulin resistance, the continual spiking and dropping of blood sugar can lead to overeating as the brain sends out hunger signals in response to low blood sugar.

PROTEIN POWER

Protein is amazing stuff—and an absolute necessity. Protein is the body's building block. It is essential in building and repairing muscle tissue, organs, and all of the connective tissues like tendons and ligaments. It contributes to the health of our skin, hair, and nails. Protein reduces cravings, balances blood sugar and helps manage weight. If you need to lose weight, it helps burn fat. If you need to gain weight, it helps build muscle. Protein also produces energy and creates antibodies to fight off infectious diseases.

Protein makes us stronger.

Fortunately, protein is also abundant. Protein can be found in almost every food source in nature. We normally think of the animal sources of protein—meat, fish, poultry, and eggs. That's because they contain much higher percentages of protein. But plants also provide protein. Beans and other legumes, nuts, grains, seeds, and vegetables all contain protein, just in smaller amounts. So, here's the question: Should we get our protein from plants or animals? If you put people on vegan and paleo diets in the same room, this is what they'll argue about. To make it more confusing, you can find science to back up both sides.

Our bodies break proteins down into 21 amino acids, 12 of which the body can manufacture on its own. Since our bodies cannot manufacture the other nine amino acids, they are considered "essential" amino acids. "Complete" proteins, such as those from animal sources, supply all of these essential amino acids. "Incomplete" proteins are generally found in plants and lack one or more of the essential amino acids. For this reason, it is important for vegetarians and vegans to consume protein from a variety of sources, such as combining grains with legumes. And some plants— quinoa for example—contain all nine essential amino acids.

So where should you get your protein from? Honestly, it's an individual issue. Listen to your body because it will let you know what it performs better on. Personally, I tend to believe fewer animal products is better, but I am not against them. I still include them in my diet, just a lot less than I used to.

The most important thing is to make sure that any animal products you eat are clean, quality proteins. It matters how the animal was raised, what it ate, how humanely it was treated, and how it was slaughtered. My family gets most of our meat from a farm that we know takes care of its animals.

Grass-fed beef is better for you. It's much leaner than conventional beef and is higher in several key nutrients, including antioxidants, vitamins, and a beneficial fat called conjugated linoleic acid (CLA). CLA has been shown to improve immune system function and has anti-inflammation benefits. Plus, grass-fed beef has about 50 percent more omega-3 fatty acids than conventional beef. That's a good thing. Oh, and it tastes better.

If you are a hunter, or know one, deer, and elk are excellent sources of protein. If you eat fish it should be wild-caught. The best eggs are farm fresh eggs laid by chickens that get to run around and be chickens. You want pasture raised eggs. (Cage free and free range are not the same thing.) Yes, they cost more, but they are so much more delicious and so much better for you. Do a little experiment, take a good pastured egg and a factory-farmed egg and crack them both in a bowl together. The yolk of the pastured egg is a much darker yellow, even almost orange at times, while the other egg is a pale yellow.

THE SKINNY ON FATS

Before carbs became "the enemy" in the 90s, fats were the pariahs of the 80's. We all saw the studies that linked high-fat diets to increased risk of heart disease, cancer, diabetes, and other problems; but those studies are beginning to come under fire. More recent studies show that sugar and refined carbs are the primary causes of heart disease. It also appears that those older studies that made fat the bad guy were funded by the sugar industry, indicating a possible conflict of interest.

The fact is that fats are an essential part of a healthy diet. Like everything else, you have to know the difference between good fats and bad fats. Good fat is necessary for producing energy, transporting fat-soluble vitamins, providing insulation, maintaining healthy skin and hair, and supplying the "essential" fat, linoleic acid. Like the amino acids, essential fatty acids are not present in the body, so you have to get them from food. And they are essential in controlling inflammation, blood clotting and brain function. (That's because your brain is 60 percent fat? That's pretty significant.)

We had a friend in Memphis whose father was a missionary in Africa. He was fluent in the local language; but as he developed some early signs of dementia he began to lose the language. Our friend consulted a naturopathic doctor and got her father on a high-fat diet—lots of avocados, coconut oil, and other good fats. In time, the signs of dementia went away and his use of the local language came back.

Our bodies also need fat to absorb certain vitamins. You may have heard the term "fat-soluble vitamins." Fat-soluble vitamins are those that dissolve in fats and oils and are absorbed along with the fats in your diet. Vitamins A, D, E and K are fat-soluble. Fat is also a great source of energy—probably one of the best. So, the bottom line—you need fats to live and thrive.

So where can you get healthy fats?

Good sources of monounsaturated fats include nuts, oils from nuts (such as almonds, macadamias, cashews), extra-virgin olive oil, avocados, flaxseed, and sesame seeds. Those are a good starting point. There are also polyunsaturated fats, which provide those essential fatty acids (EFAs) our bodies don't manufacture on their own—like Omega-3 and Omega-6 EFAs. Omega-3 is an amazingly healthy fat found in fish, nuts, seeds, avocados, olives, algae, green plants, coconut oil, and extra-virgin olive oil. These fats have been proven to reduce diabetes, heart disease, cancer and dementia. Omega-6 EFAs come from grains, vegetables oils, poultry and eggs.

Most of us already get plenty of Omega-6 EFAs in our diet, but we're lacking in Omega-3s. Omega-6 is found in abundance in processed foods, especially those that contain soybean oil or palm oil. It is also found in higher percentages in the meats of grain-fed animals—another reason to eat grass-fed meat. Ideally, we should be getting a 2:1 ratio, about two parts

Omega-6 to one part Omega-3. Most people today get somewhere between 10:1 and 25:1.[21]

SUPERFOODS

You may have heard the term "superfood," but never really knew what that means. Superfoods are just that—super-foods. If you are looking for an easy way to feel great, lose weight and function better, start adding more superfoods to your diet.

What are superfoods? They are the most nutrient-dense foods on the planet. In a nutshell, they "are whole foods that have not been processed and go beyond basic nutrition. They are foods that contain various combinations of vitamins, minerals, or antioxidants that help prevent disease and sickness while promoting outstanding health benefits."[22] In his book *Superfoods: The Food and Medicine of the Future*, David Wolfe breaks them into superfoods and super-herbs. Superfoods, he says, "include foods that have a dozen or more unique properties, not just one or two."[23] For example, the goji berry is a source of complete protein, and contains antioxidants, over twenty trace minerals, and other compounds that boost your immune system, cleanse your liver, and have anti-aging effects. Superherbs he defined as "herbs that have super tonic and adaptogenic properties as well as many other unique gifts."[24] Adaptogens are natural compounds that assist the adrenal system in regulating hormones and managing stress.

So, which superfoods should you be eating? That's a great question. Unfortunately, the answer is not so simple. Darin Olien is world-renowned as "The Ingredient Hunter." You may have seen him featured in *O Magazine* a few years ago. Darin advised, "First, we need to understand the proper uses of superfoods. They are a way of bridging a gap. They're not cure-alls. They should fit in somewhere between our normal food intake and our nutritional supplements and medicines."[25]

There are, of course, lots of ways to get superfoods into your diet, but first, it will probably help to know what they are. David Wolfe's Top 10 Superfoods include the following: goji berries, cacao, maca, bee products (such as honey and royal jelly), spirulina, AFA blue-green algae, marine phytoplankton, aloe vera, hempseed, and coconuts. He also lists açai, camu came berry, chlorella, Incan berries, kelp, noni, and yacon as "honorable mentions."[26] Steven Pratt, a medical doctor and author of *SuperFoods RX: Fourteen Foods That Will Change Your Life*, lists a few more common foods: beans, blueberries, broccoli, oats, oranges, pumpkin, salmon, edamame, spinach, tea (green or black), tomatoes, turkey, walnuts, and yogurt.

Next you need to get over your food biases. Our taste buds adapt, so taste is based on habit and familiarity. If you haven't tried it, you don't know if you like it or not. Or perhaps you had it once, but it wasn't prepared the right way. For example, I don't like mushy broccoli, but I love nice, crisp lightly steamed broccoli.

Plus, there are also plenty of ways to "sneak" them into your diet—like mixing them into smoothies. You can make them yourself at home, and you can find recipes all over the internet.

You could very easily throw spirulina, blueberries, coconut, or honey into a smoothie in the morning. You can add walnuts to your steel-cut oatmeal in the morning and sweeten it with a teaspoon of honey or dark maple syrup. You can make your own salad dressings with apple cider vinegar, honey, or dark maple syrup. Our favorite salad dressing is the Creamy Garlic recipe from the Ultimate Reset. If you need more ideas, a quick online search will lead you to plenty of options.

You can do it. I have faith in you.

WHY ORGANIC?

When it comes to food, clean doesn't mean "not-dirty." Ironically, dirt is probably the cleanest thing our food comes into contact with. In fact, plants need dirt. No, when it comes to food, clean means free of harmful chemicals such as pesticides, herbicides, and petroleum-based fertilizers. Clean means organic or naturally grown.

But doesn't organic food cost more? It does, but that reminds me of an old saying: "Better to pay your grocer now than your doctor later." Keep in mind, the doctor bills would be the least of your problems. The real problem is all the damage those toxins can do to your body. So, you could feel sick, tired, and half dead, but you'll still have to pay up. On the other hand, you can invest in yourself now and be vibrant and healthy. It's totally your call.

The problem with pesticides and herbicides is that they are good at their jobs—they're killers. They kill off the insects that eat plants and destroy crops. They kill the weeds and other plants that choke off whatever you're trying to grow. They are poisons and toxins—and that's the problem.

As Dr. Mercola observed, "It should be revealing that one commonly used type of pesticide, organophosphates, were first developed as nerve gas during World War II."[27] If you think it will kill an insect, do you really think it won't have any effect on you? Part of the problem is that the EPA approved and registered many of today's chemicals long before the harmful side effects were known. Now, those effects are coming to light. For instance, a 2004 study published by the National Institutes of Health showed an increased risk of cancer among 17,000 children living on farms where pesticide use had increased. *Kids on the Frontline*, a report released in 2016 by the Pesticide Action Network, reflects a rigorous assessment of dozens of independent studies documenting links between pesticide exposure and children's health harms. "The science linking agricultural pesticides to childhood health harms — particularly leukemia, brain tumors and developmental disorders — has grown increasingly strong."[28] Other studies have shown an increased risk of several kinds of cancer, leukemia, lymphoma, Parkinson's disease, ALS, fetal birth defects, asthma and other respiratory ailments, diabetes, ADHD, and even an increased risk of death due to heart disease.[29] [30]

And, yes, I am aware of the Stanford University study that claimed there is no "meaningful" difference in nutrient content between organic and non-organic produce. But it's not just about the nutrient content. No scientist has ever demonstrated that these chemicals are good for us. But here's something else . . . that very same Stanford study found that organic strawberries had higher levels of vitamin C and that organic produce contained more phenols than non-organic produce. Phenols are compounds believed to help prevent cancer. The Stanford study, while convenient, fails to overcome the numerous other studies that demonstrate significant differences between organic and non-organic produce.

But I get it—organic produce costs more. So, if you can't buy all organic produce, it helps to prioritize. Every year, the Environmental Working Group (EWG) puts out a list of their "Dirty Dozen" and "Clean Fifteen." Its "Dirty Dozen" list singles out produce with the highest pesticide loads. For 2016, that list included strawberries, apples, nectarines, peaches, celery, grapes, cherries, spinach, tomatoes, sweet bell peppers, cherry tomatoes, and cucumbers. The EWG recently expanded their Dirty Dozen list with a "Plus" category to highlight two types of food that contain trace levels of highly hazardous pesticides. "Two American food crops—leafy greens and hot peppers—are of special concern for public health because residue tests conducted by the U.S. Department of Agriculture have found these foods laced with particularly toxic pesticides."[31]

The "Clean Fifteen" identifies conventionally grown fruits and vegetables that tend to test low for pesticide residues. For 2016, those were avocados, sweet corn, pineapples, cabbage, frozen sweet peas, onions, asparagus, mangoes, papayas, kiwis, eggplant, honeydew melon, grapefruit, cantaloupe, and cauliflower.

CALORIES VS. CALORIES

For years, we've seen an enormous focus on calories. Some people count calories, while others cut calories or add calories. But do we even know what a calorie is?

In simplest terms, calories are a measure of energy—generally the amount of energy contained in a particular food. This is important because our bodies need a certain amount of energy (i.e. calories) every day.

But if you eat too many calories day after day, your body will begin to store the extra energy in the form of fat. For example, if you consume 500 calories a day more than you burn off, you will gain about a pound a week. Likewise, if you eat too few calories your body may think you are trying to starve it and may begin storing energy for later use, again in the form of fat.

So how many calories a day should you consume? That depends on a lot of things: height, weight, activity level, body composition, and genetics just to name a few. But it's also the wrong question to be asking because not all calories are created equal.

A calorie is a unit of measurement, like a pound or kilogram. A pound is always a pound. A ton of feathers and a ton of bricks weigh exactly the same, but if you drop them both off the top of a tall building, you'll get very different results. Which one would you rather be standing under? See what I mean?

For example, a typical 20-ounce soda has about 240 calories. Compare that to 240 calories of broccoli—about 7.5 cups. Do you see where this is going? What's the soda going to do to your health? It's going to wreck it in more ways than you can imagine. And the broccoli? Assuming you could eat 7.5 cups in one sitting, those 240 calories would do something very different. Let's take a look at how this all plays out in your body.

The 240 calories from the 20-ounce soda all come from sugar. According to the label, it contains 65 grams of sugar (that's more than 16 teaspoons!) in the form of high fructose corn syrup.[32] It also contains caffeine and phosphoric acid, which causes osteoporosis. It contains no vitamins, no minerals and no fiber.

When you drink the soda, your gut quickly absorbs the fiber-free sugars and your blood sugar immediately begins to spike. According to Dr. Hyman, this begins "a domino effect of high insulin and a cascade of hormonal responses that kicks bad biochemistry into gear."[33] The high insulin increases storage of belly fat, and increases inflammation throughout your body. It also raises your triglycerides and bad cholesterol while lowering your good cholesterol. It raises blood pressure, lowers testosterone in men, and contributes to infertility in women. It also causes a fatty liver, increases cortisol (the stress hormone) and causes diabetes, cancer and dementia. And we're just getting started.[34]

The insulin blocks your body's appetite control hormone, leptin, you become leptin resistant and your body never gets the signal that you're full. On the contrary, your brain thinks your body is starving. Then the sugar releases massive amounts of the feel-good hormone dopamine into your brain, triggering your pleasure-based reward system. Now you're addicted and you have a nearly overwhelming drive to consume more sugar.

Are you seeing a vicious cycle forming? I won't even go into the potential problems you could run into from the ingredients sourced from genetically engineered crops or GMO's they admit they contain.[35] The 240 calories in the soda you drank are there, but they are empty calories, meaning they are completely devoid of any real nutritional value. They are, however, in the words of Dr. Hyman, "full of trouble."[36]

Not to mention the fact that the super sweetness of the soda hijacks your taste buds, so you lose the ability to enjoy naturally sweet foods like blueberries or other fruit—the foods God intended to satisfy your sweet cravings. We'll get to that a little more in a bit.

Now for the broccoli. For starters, the calorie makeup is much more balanced. A cup of raw broccoli contains approximately 46 grams of carbohydrates, 20 grams of protein, and 2 grams of fat. It also contains nearly 19 grams of dietary fiber. Of the 46 grams of carbs, only 1.5 are from sugar—the equivalent of only 0.375 teaspoons. Like all non-starchy vegetables, broccoli is an extremely low glycemic food with a glycemic index of 15 (anything below 55 is considered low). The high-fiber, low-sugar carbohydrates are digested slowly and therefore don't lead to blood sugar and insulin spikes. Because there is no blood sugar and insulin spike, there is no fatty liver and hormonal chaos. Your brain gets the signal that your body is full, so you probably wouldn't be able to eat the whole 7.5 cups anyway. Nothing bad happens at all. Quite the opposite in fact. Broccoli is rich in vitamins and minerals, including folate and magnesium, which is essential for absorbing calcium, which it also contains. It also contains those powerful phytonutrients that help heal and detoxify your body. In Dr. Hyman's words, you get the "many extra benefits that optimize metabolism, lower cholesterol, reduce inflammation, and boost detoxification. The phytonutrients in broccoli (glucosinolates) boost your liver's ability to detoxify environmental chemicals, and the flavonoid kaempferol is a powerful anti-inflammatory. Broccoli also contains high levels of vitamin C and folate, which protect against cancer and heart disease. The glucosinolates and sulphorophanes in broccoli change the expression of your genes to help balance your sex hormones, reducing breast and other cancers."[37]

I'm sure you get the picture, the broccoli creates health, while the soda destroys it. Same calories—very different effects. Some calories, like sugar, are addictive and destructive, while others, like broccoli, are healing. Some calories lead to weight gain, while others boost your metabolism. That's because food is more than just calories. Every single thing you eat or drink, every bite, every sip, contains information that is passed on to your body in the form of coded instructions—instructions that will either create health or disease.

A calorie is not just a calorie. It really is a case of quality over quantity. You have the power to choose life or death, health or disease, by what you choose to eat. Which will you choose?

ADDICTED

I would be negligent if I left this chapter without talking about our food addictions. Does that sound harsh or like a hyperbole? Well, what else would you call it? Why else would so many of us consume foods that we know are not good for us? Why would we choose to be obese? Why would we be so eager to eat foods that we know can—and will—destroy our health and leave us with a sense of guilt and shame?

We're hooked.

Do you remember our earlier discussion about how the food industry—or as Dr. Mark Hyman calls it, the industrial food complex—has created these hyper-processed, hyper-palatable, highly addictive foods that are sabotaging our brain chemistry, our waistlines, and our health? If not, here's a refresher: "The science of food addiction is clearer now than ever before. A powerful study recently published in the *American Journal of Clinical Nutrition* proves that higher-sugar, higher-glycemic foods are addictive in the same way as cocaine and heroin."[38]

Yep, sugar is eight times as addictive as cocaine. On the surface, that seems like a bit of a stretch. But if you look around you, what you see indicates that it's probably not. For example, ever seen a kid craving candy or cake or pie. I have. They act just like a drug addict.

In 2009, Dr. Serge H. Ahmed published "Is Sugar as Addictive as Cocaine?" in the journal *Food and Addiction*. The study proved that the answer was "yes." Dr. Ahmed found that when rats were offered cocaine or sugar (in the form of artificially sweetened water) they always went for the sugar, even if they had previously been addicted to cocaine.[39]

Let that sink in for a second. The rats preferred the equivalent of a soda to cocaine. And it's not just sodas that are the problem. Take a look at your favorite energy drink or sport drink or tea. And you wonder why it's so hard to kick your sweet tooth.

Well, we should just switch to artificial sweeteners, right? Wrong! You'd be better off with real sugar—high-fructose corn syrup doesn't really count, but it's still better for you than the chemical nightmares that are artificial sweeteners. For starters, artificial sweeteners like aspartame (NutraSweet), sucralose (Splenda), and acesulfame potassium actually make you fat and cause type 2 diabetes.

Say what? How is that possible since they have no calories. If calories were all that mattered, that might be the case; but we know better now, don't we? Don't let the food industry fool you. There is no magic alternative to sugar when it comes to sweeteners. Artificial sweeteners increase cravings, weight gain, and Type 2 diabetes. Plus, they are addictive. Additional side effects can include: headaches, gastrointestinal problems; seizures, dizziness and migraines; blurred vision; and allergic reactions.

Dr. Hyman cited a study of 66,118 women conducted over a fourteen-year period that was published in the *American Journal of Clinical Nutrition* (and supported by numerous other studies) that showed some rather frightening facts about the consumption of diet drinks and artificial sweeteners.

- Diet sodas raised the risk of diabetes more than sugar-sweetened sodas.
- Women who drank one twelve-ounce diet soda a week had a 33 percent increased risk of type 2 diabetes, and women who drank one twenty-ounce soda a week had a 66 percent increased risk.
- Women who drank diet sodas drank twice as much as those who drank sugar-sweetened sodas because artificial sweeteners are more addictive than regular sugar.
- The average diet soda drinker consumes three diet drinks a day.
- Artificial sweeteners are hundreds to thousands of times sweeter than regular sugar, activating our genetically programmed preference for sweetness more than any other substance.
- Artificial sweeteners trick your metabolism into thinking sugar is on its way. This causes your body to pump out insulin, the fat-storage hormone, which leads to more belly fat.

- Artificial sweeteners confuse and slow down your metabolism, so you burn fewer calories every day. They make you hungrier and cause you to crave even more sugar and starchy carbs, such as bread and pasta.
- In animal studies, the rats that consumed artificial sweeteners ate more food, their metabolic fire (or thermogenesis) slowed down, and they put on 14 percent more body fat in just two weeks—even if they ate fewer total calories than the rats that ate regular sugar-sweetened food.[40]

Bottom line: sugar is a treat that should be enjoyed occasionally. The American Heart Association recommends limiting sugar intake to no more than half of your daily discretionary calorie allowance: No more than 100 calories per day for women (about 6 teaspoons) and no more than 150 calories per day for men (9 teaspoons).[41] Again, it's your call.

And sugar is only part of the problem. We're addicted to the chemically engineered, highly palatable, nutrient poor, calorie dense, toxic nightmares that are processed foods. That is not God's design for us. When we eat the foods He created for us to eat, we are healthy, vibrant and strong—not addicted.

AVOID AT ALL COST

Okay, maybe "avoid at all cost" is a bit much, but there are foods you should definitely avoid as much as possible. Do you recall the quote from Dr. Wigmore: "The food you eat can be either the safest and most powerful form of medicine, or the slowest form of poison?" I'm assuming you'd rather not poison yourself if you can help it—even if it does happen slowly over time. Would it be helpful to know which foods are the worst offenders?

If you just stick to the rule of eating real food, this isn't a problem. Real food heals. In a nutshell, if you avoid processed foods, this won't be an issue for you. But just to be thorough, let's take a look at a few reasons to avoid processed foods. (Oh, and don't be fooled by health claims on the package—there is plenty of junk "health" food out there. And you have to be extremely careful with performance supplements.) Here are a few things to watch out for.

The term "processed" can be confusing, so let's clarify what we are talking about. There is whole food, meaning single ingredient food. Think apples, broccoli, tomatoes, kale, and such. I like what Michael Pollen said, "If it came from a plant, eat it; if it was made in a plant, don't."[42]

By "processed" foods, I mean foods that have been chemically processed and made primarily from refined ingredients and artificial substances and "franken-chemicals." These foods make up more than 60 percent of the American diet. It's time to take back our food supply. Here are some of the most toxic things to look for as you learn to read labels.

We've already talked about the importance of eating organic as much as possible, so you already know that you don't want food that has been sprayed with chemicals. If I offered you an apple I had just drenched with bug spray and weed killer, you would look at me like I was crazy. You wouldn't come near it—even if I told you to just rinse it off. So don't eat produce that someone else did that to. Common sense, right?

You can also add chicken, fish, and beef. Those are single ingredient foods. But you want to make sure that your chicken and beef and eggs are pasture raised, grass-fed, and antibiotic free. Your fish should be wild caught. Again, we want our food to be grown/raised the way God intended it to be.

Nut butters, if they are single ingredient, are also fine. If you buy peanut butter, the ingredients should read: peanuts. Maybe a little sea salt. Not salt—salt refers to processed, refined salt. Sea salts and Himalayan salt are minimally processed and contain a wealth of trace minerals and electrolytes that are easily assimilated by your body. That's it. No added oils or sugars. You should have to stir it when you open it up at home.

Oh, and just because the FDA says something is safe, it doesn't mean it is. It's scary to see the list of products that were once deemed "FDA Approved" or "Generally Recognized As Safe" but were later pulled from market when shown to be downright dangerous. It's a personal decision; but for me, it's not worth risking my family's health.

Sugar. We've talked a little bit about how addictive and harmful sugar is, especially high fructose corn syrup (HFCS). There are at least 61 names sugar hides behind. Sugar, sucrose, HFCS, corn syrup, barley malt, dextrose, maltose, rice syrup, beet sugar, fruit juice, and evaporated cane juice just to name a few. The average Americans eats up to 60 pounds of high fructose corn syrup a year. Sixty pounds!!

You may have seen the ad that says that HFCS is the same as any other sugar. Did you happen to catch who sponsored that ad? The corn lobby. Did you know that they also funded the study they quoted.[43] Ever heard of the fox guarding the hen house?

HFCS is in almost everything, so it's the one to really avoid. It contains contaminants, like mercury, that the FDA neither measures nor regulates. It increases the level of triglycerides in your blood, as well as fat-storing hormones. It has also been linked to non-alcoholic fatty liver disease and cirrhosis of the liver. Time to go on a sugar detox.

Artificial Sweeteners. Again, we have already covered this a little bit. When the low-carb craze hit, the food industry offered us a sweet, low or no-calorie alternative. It was a sweet deception. I can't stress enough how bad this stuff is for you. If you see aspartame, sucralose, saccharin, or acesulfame potassium on the label, put it down and run away.

Artificial Colors. Chemicals like Red No. 40 and 3, Yellow No. 5, Green No. 6 and Blue No. 1 and 2 make food look prettier. Sort of like lipstick on a pig—but it's toxic lipstick. Artificial food colorings have known side effects including hyperactivity, chromosomal damage, migraines, cancer, asthma, and heart issues[44]. Europe has actually banned several of these chemicals because they found links to ADHD, cancer and other health conditions. American food manufactures actually changed the ingredients for safer coloring like beet juice in place of red dye in order to sell their products in the EU. But they still sell us the toxic versions.[45] You might want to skip these.

Sodas and Sports Drinks. Step away from the soft drink!! Twelve ounces of soda contains approximately 150 calories and 10 teaspoons of sugar, usually in the form of high fructose corn syrup. That's more than the maximum daily sugar intake recommended by the American Heart Association. Sodas also have anywhere from 30 to 55 mg of caffeine and are loaded with artificial food colors and sulphites. Sulphites are preservatives added to many foods that can cause symptoms such as wheezing, fainting and irritation of the digestive system in those who are susceptible. Not to mention the fact that it is so acidic you can use it to clean off your car battery terminals. Imagine what that does to your gut! I can't think of any good reason to ever drink it. The diet varieties are even worse, as they are filled with harmful artificial sweeteners like aspartame and sucralose.

Studies have linked soda to osteoporosis, obesity, tooth decay and heart disease,[46] yet the average American drinks an estimated 50 gallons of soft drinks each year. Plus, drinking all that sugar will likely suppress your appetite for healthy foods, which paves the way for nutrient deficiencies.

So-called "sports drinks" are also notoriously high in sugar, and the acid erodes the teeth even more than soda. They also have high levels of sodium, which increases your risk of stroke and heart disease.[47] Unless you're a high-level athlete engaged in intense and extended workouts, stay away. Even then, you're better off with water.[48]

Hydrogenated Oils. These oils have had hydrogen added to them to extend shelf life. You most often find them in fried foods and baked goods.

The problem is, adding hydrogen to oil tends to produce a trans-fat, a particularly evil kind of fat that causes a number of health problems including cardiovascular disease and diabetes. You don't want it.

Refined, Enriched, or White Grains. Grains aren't naturally white. When a whole grain is refined, all of the nutrients end up being stripped away. That's why they "enrich" them to try to add some of the nutrients back in. It doesn't work very well. Without the nutrients and fiber of a whole grain, these refined grains are basically a delivery system for sugar. Your body converts white flour to sugar and spikes your insulin levels just like a teaspoon of pure sugar—and we know what that does to you. Put it down.

Sodium Nitrates And Sodium Nitrites. No, I'm not being redundant. Those are two different chemicals—preservatives most often found in processed meats like hot dogs, lunch meat, and bacon. They are believed to be carcinogenic (cancer causing) and may also lead to metabolic syndrome and diabetes. Livestrong.com warns, "According to the American Medical Association, a diet high in sodium nitrites may lead to a health condition called methemoglobinemia, which is the inability of your red blood cells to transport oxygen throughout your body. This condition causes respiratory problems and can be fatal."[49] The good news is you can find amazing organic meats that are free of these toxins. But Dr. Axe suggests avoiding processed meats altogether and instead choosing, "organic, freshly prepared meats, such as grass-fed beef, organic, free-range chicken and wild-caught fish."[50]

Canned Tomatoes. Tomatoes are healthy, right? Fresh, organic locally-grown tomatoes are. Canned tomatoes can actually be quite toxic. They often contain a nasty cocktail of preservatives. What's worse, the lining of most canned goods contains bisphenol-A (BPA). BPA is a synthetic compound that mimics estrogen in the body. Dr. Mercola says it "is an endocrine disrupter, which means it mimics or interferes with your body's hormones and 'disrupts' your endocrine system."[51] BPA has been linked to a number of health concerns, including structural damage to your brain; changes in gender-specific behavior and abnormal sexual behavior; hyperactivity; increased aggressiveness and impaired learning; early puberty; stimulation of mammary gland development; disrupted reproductive cycles; ovarian dysfunction and infertility; increased fat formation and risk of obesity; stimulation of prostate cancer cells; increased prostate size and decreased sperm production; and altered immune function.[52] You're better off choosing organic tomatoes packed in glass jars, or finding a brand that has a BPA free liner.

Monosodium Glutamate (MSG). MSG is a flavor enhancer most often associated with Chinese food, but it is found in almost all commercially prepared and packaged foods. In 1959, the U.S. Food and Drug Administration labeled MSG as "Generally Recognized as Safe" (GRAS), and it has remained that way ever since. Interestingly, 10 years later a condition known as "Chinese Restaurant Syndrome" began to pop up in medical literature, describing symptoms such as headaches, skin flushing, and sweating that people experienced after eating MSG. Today that syndrome is more appropriately called "MSG Symptom Complex." According to Dr. Mercola, "One of the best overviews of the very real dangers of MSG comes from Dr. Russell Blaylock, a board-certified neurosurgeon and author of *Excitotoxins: The Taste that Kills.*" In it he explains that MSG is an excitotoxin, which means it overexcites your cells to the point of damage or death, causing brain damage to varying degrees –and potentially even triggering or worsening learning disabilities, Alzheimer's disease, Parkinson's disease, Lou Gehrig's disease and more." [53] In his book, *In Bad Taste: The MSG Symptom Complex*, Dr. George Schwartz demonstrated that the increase in cases of ADD, ADHD, asthma, and teenage depression are the result of the increase in consumption of MSG.[54] Doesn't sound that safe, after all.

To be honest, this is just a starter list. I could go on for pages and pages, but I have a better idea. Just eat real, clean, whole foods, and you won't have to worry about any of these.

SUPPLEMENTS

I am frequently asked about supplements, including protein shakes and bars, vitamins, probiotics, and pre- and post-workout supplements. A couple of months ago one of the youth at church walked up to me drinking a protein shake and said, "Aren't you proud of me? I'm drinking a protein shake." Considering that it would have been much easier for her to just eat the pizza and junk that everyone else was eating, I was extremely proud of her and told her so. Then I asked what brand it was and if she would mind if I looked at the label. "Does it matter?" she asked. Absolutely. I had her pull up the label on my iPad and we looked at it together. I showed her all of the ingredients listed that were not good. After doing her own research, she has since switched to another brand. Lesson learned.

All of the rules we have been talking about apply to supplements as well. You want to make sure that they are as clean and natural as possible— preferably from whole food sources. They should be free of artificial ingredients like artificial sweeteners and colors. Watch out for excess levels of caffeine and niacin. Beware of anything that makes your heart race. I prefer vegan proteins or organic grass-fed whey. They are out there, you just have to look for them. Again, you will pay more for clean supplements, but you're worth it. I'm the kind of person who researches and tests everything, and will only recommend products I trust. Any product that I talk about or link to on social media or my blog is one that I have personally used and trust.

Whatever you choose, make sure you have done your homework.

TEARING DOWN STRONGHOLDS

Addiction is a vicious cycle, and food addiction is no different. We eat bad foods because we crave them, yet we crave bad foods because we eat them. We have to break the addiction cycle. We have to tear down the strongholds that the enemy has established in our lives and against our health.

Strongholds are built on lies—the lies the enemy whispers in our ears, the lies others have spoken over us, and the lies we tell ourselves. From the moment we first agree with these lies, they begin to build our prison. The first step in tearing them down is to recognize this for the spiritual battle that it is. Fortunately, "The weapons we fight with are not the weapons of the world. On the contrary, they have divine power to demolish strongholds" (2 Corinthians 10:4 NIV).

Our first weapon is "the sword of the Spirit, which is the word of God" (Ephesians 6:17 NIV). That is where this book came from, my journey through God's Word and seeing all the wisdom it contains about health and our bodies. Our second weapon is prayer. Here is a prayer that I encourage you to pray. Say it out loud because there is something about hearing the prayer in your own voice. And the words don't have to be exact, so just pray what's in your heart:

Lord Jesus, thank You for creating me and loving me. Thank You for coming to give your life for mine and bringing me into a right relationship with the Father. Thank you for forgiving me of my sins and granting to me your righteousness. Thank You that You understand my temptations and frustrations and that You have promised to always provide a way for me to overcome them. I recognize that I cannot do this on my own and acknowledge that I am powerless to change my deeply ingrained habits without You. I need You to heal me physically and emotionally and spiritually. Father, forgive me. I confess that I have been offering myself over to sin and have become enslaved by it. I repent of my sins and I renounce them in Jesus' name. I renounce the ways I have allowed my appetites and desires to become idols. I renounce the ways I have turned to food for comfort instead of turning to You. I sanctify my body to Jesus Christ and commit to glorify Him in my body. I dedicate my life to You. I offer my body as a living sacrifice to You, Jesus, including all my appetites and desires. Cover me with Your blood, cleanse me of my sins and wash me white as snow. I am completely Yours.

Holy Spirit, search me and know me. Test me and know my heart and mind. Show me areas in my health and fitness that may be offensive to You. Show me where I have listened to the lies of the enemy and made agreements with him. I renounce those agreements now. Satan has no authority over me, nor does any other foul thing, or any person. I am Yours, Jesus, and Yours alone. I renounce the agreement that I am alone, for You are always with me (Matthew 28:20). I am surrounded by a great cloud of witnesses (Hebrews 12:1). I renounce the agreement that I am powerless, for I can do all things through Your strength (Philippians 4:13). I renounce every agreement with shame and guilt, for there is therefore now no condemnation for those who are in Christ Jesus (Romans 8:1). Holy Spirit, show me what to pray and intercede for me on my behalf (Romans 8:26).

I bring the blood of Christ, right here, right now against every stronghold in my life and against the spirits behind them. I banish these enemies from my life now—from my body, my soul, and my spirit. I claim the promise, "Resist the devil, and he will flee from you" (James 4:7 ESV). I resist the devil and command him and all evil spirits to flee in the authority of the Lord Jesus Christ and in His name.

Father, forgive me for allowing my desire for unhealthy food and drinks to control me. Forgive me for allowing fear and complacency a place in my heart. Forgive me for giving resignation and the spirit of defeat and shame a place in my life. Forgive me for not allowing You complete lordship over my life. I am Yours— body, soul and spirit. Take Your rightful place in my life now, Lord Jesus. Set me free from all that has enslaved me. I plead Your blood over my life and I break every chain and every place I have given my enemies control. It is for freedom that You have set me free (Galatians 5:1) Sanctify me completely, and may my "whole soul and spirit and body be kept blameless at the coming of our Lord Jesus Christ" (1 Thessalonians 5:23). Even so, come, Lord Jesus.

Jesus, I need Your healing touch. I come to You now to be renewed in You, to be restored in You, to receive from You the grace and mercy I so desperately need this day and every day. Lord Jesus, You have been sent "to bind up the brokenhearted, to proclaim freedom for the captives and release from darkness for the prisoners, to proclaim the year of the Lord's favor and the day of vengeance of our God (Isaiah 61:1-2). Jesus, come and heal my broken heart, set me free from this captivity and open my eyes to the light of Your truth. Lord, grant me Your favor and bring Your vengeance against those who oppose Your will for my life. Lord, You came to comfort all who mourn, and provide for those who grieve in Zion—to bestow on them a crown of beauty instead of ashes, the oil of joy instead of mourning, and a garment of praise instead of a spirit of despair (Isaiah 61:2-3). Jesus, I ask You to do this for me now. Comfort me where I am hurting, bestow on me a crown of beauty instead of ashes, anoint me with the oil of joy instead of mourning, dress me in a garment of praise instead a spirit of despair. Behold old things have passed away; I am a new creation in Christ (2 Corinthians 5:17).

In Jesus' name, amen.

How does that feel? As powerful as the Word of God and prayer are, they won't do you much good until you take action. Tearing down strongholds is hard work, and we have to do our part. I am indebted to John Eldredge and Ransomed Heart ministries for teaching me how to pray with power. It has dramatically changed my life. Whatever you are struggling with, name it and be specific. For example, "I renounce the agreement that I am fat; I renounce the agreement that I can't help myself; I renounce the agreement that You don't care about my body." You will find that the more you pray like this, the more you will begin to see yourself as Jesus sees you and the more you will feel empowered to create lasting change.

OVERCOMING MY ADDICTIONS

When it comes to breaking food addictions, you probably need to do some sort of elimination diet or detox diet. There are several good ones out there—just make sure you choose one focused on a diet of whole, fresh, clean foods and completely natural supplements. My first experience with one of these began in March of 2012. I was invited to participate in a test group for a 21-day detox program that was divided into three week-long phases. It was a food based elimination detox with natural supplements to help maximize results.

I had allowed myself a little too much leeway on my diet the previous Thanksgiving and Christmas season. Plus, we had just returned from a vacation where I had indulged a little too much. As part of the test group, the company paid for us to have our blood work done before and after the detox.

I have to admit, I was nervous going in. There were foods in the meal plan that I hated, including cucumbers and tomatoes. There were foods I had never tried—like kale. And there were foods I had never even heard of. What the heck is tempeh, anyway?

I remember that on my first trip to Whole Foods I had printed off my shopping list for the week, but I kept needing to ask someone what things were and where to find them. Mind you, this is four full years after my transformation. I was eating clean—I thought. I had lost weight. I had been in the best shape of my life, but remember this is not about appearances or weight.

In the first phase, you start to reclaim your body. You are beginning the process of healing from the inside out. Those first seven days were both some of the hardest and some of the best. The food was absolutely amazing! These are recipes our family still uses today because everyone loves them. I also discovered some new loves, like the Roasted Root Medley and the Zucchini Cashew soup. I discovered the power of having a huge healthy green salad for lunch almost every day.

Those who were not vegan began weaning themselves off of animal protein. The first week we still had eggs, salmon, chicken and yogurt as part of the meal plan.

I could go on and on about how great the food was. By about the third day I was even starting to like cucumbers and tomatoes. When I told my mom about that she asked who I was and what I had done with her son! Everything started to have so much flavor—like my taste buds were coming alive for the first time. I remember having a fruit bowl for breakfast on Day 4 and that first bite was like an explosion of tastes. God's candy! Who knew?

So, what was the hard part? The process of detoxing. I had headaches the first two days. Day 3 felt pretty normal, though I was starting to get a little absent-minded. Day 4 was a Saturday, and it's the reason most people started the detox on a Wednesday. Day 4 and 5 of a detox are often the days that you just want to lay in bed—and if you can, you should. Your body is working overtime to flush out toxins and heal. When Day 6 rolled around on Monday, I was amazed at how much more energy I already had. I bounced out of bed raring to go.

From the start of the second phase on, the meal plan was completely vegan. We also added a detox supplement for this phase. No worries, this was not a harsh detox, and there was no need to stay close to a bathroom. It just helped improve liver function so our body could eliminate toxins more efficiently. It also supports colon function. It was a bit on the chalky side so I had to take it more like a shot and chase it with lots of water. Sometimes, you just have to take your medicine.

Something else got released this week—my emotions. About halfway through I noticed that I was highly emotional. I would well up with emotions and sometimes the littlest things would bring me to tears. I asked the doctors and moderators of the group if this was normal. Apparently, it's not uncommon for people to release toxic emotions and drop negative habits during this phase. The strongholds were coming down, and I began to understand that this is about so much more than just food.

During the last phase we focused on restoring our gut health. We eliminated grains and were eating primarily fruits and vegetables. It was the hardest week food wise, but you start to feel amazing! The second day, Day 16 overall, we were out shopping, and I could smell a steakhouse nearby. It smelled remarkable, and I really started craving a steak or a cheeseburger—but the urge passed pretty quickly.

During this final phase, we also added a powerful probiotic to add healthy microbes back into our newly scrubbed digestive tract and restore our microbiome. The importance of this step cannot be overemphasized.

At the end of the 21 days, I felt 20 years younger. I had so much energy, it was incredible. I was sharper and more focused mentally. My eyes were clear and sparkled. My skin looked younger. A friend who was in the test group with me said that all of her cellulite had vanished. I too noticed that my skin looked and felt younger and I had shed 18 pounds and 3.5 inches off my waist.

But those are just the visible effects. What went on inside my body was even more amazing. I had my blood work done again and showed the results to my doctor. He was absolutely floored and said he had never seen results like this in such a short time. I did in three weeks what would take most people months—and would never get done with pharmaceuticals. My total cholesterol dropped, while my good cholesterol went up. My blood glucose dropped from 103 down to 87. And here's what really floored me: I had been suffering from low testosterone, but in just three weeks, my testosterone increased from 346 to 493! That's a huge leap in the right direction.

What was really odd to me was that I had lost any cravings for meat. I didn't have meat for another month or so. I really didn't miss it.

Every few months I do a maintenance detox when I began to feel the need. Once you've experienced what "clean" feels like you become more aware of how food and your environment affect you. I detox once or twice a year because it's a great way to just reboot and make sure I'm always at my best. My plan is to continue eating like Phase 1 long term. It's simple. It's a variety of fresh, clean, whole foods. It's delicious! People ask me all the time if I miss this or that food. The truth is when I'm eating this way, I don't.

TO THE POINT

Okay, so let's summarize . . .

We know that we should eat healthier, the way God intended for us to eat. In the Bible, God gave us instructions to distinguish between food that was edible and "food" that He never intended for us to eat. When God gave those rules to Moses, the only issue was which animals were clean and unclean. We know now that the flesh of unclean, inedible animals has more toxins and health risks. The New Testament introduced a new issue—food sacrificed to idols. Yes, we have freedom, but the rule never changed. We know this because in Revelation, the last book of the Bible and the final word, Jesus told two of the early churches, Pergamum and Thyatira, that one of the things He has against them is that they tolerate those who teach God's people "to sin by eating food offered to idols" (2:14, see also 2:20).

So, here's the question, what would God consider unclean or inedible today? If you consider that God's desire is to keep us healthy, that answer should be pretty obvious. Everything that does not nourish and heal is an unclean food. It's much easier to focus on the clean list. The things that God intended for food are easily identified. They are either plants that grew from the ground or in the water or animals that ate those plants. You find them along the periphery of your grocery store or at your local farmer's market.

The hardest part for most people is going to be the social pressure to conform. I get that, I really do. I've faced it. I've been at the small groups and pot-lucks and parties where people who know I am trying to eat clean offer me all sorts of "treats." But they aren't treats to me. That's not how I see them. I see them for what they are — something that is going to taste really good going down, but turn on me when it gets into my system. And actually, once you've been eating really clean for a couple of weeks, they really don't taste as good either.

Then there is that other thing—the "do not be conformed to the pattern of this world" thing. Rather, we are to be transformed by the renewing our mind (Romans 12:2). "Renew your mind" sounds awfully close to "change the way you think about something," which is the definition of repentance. We repent when we line our way of thinking up with God's. "Then you will be able to test and approve what God's will is—his good, pleasing and perfect will" (Romans 12:2 NIV).

We are supposed to be "salt and light." We are called to be holy, which means "set apart." In *The Pursuit of Holiness*, Jerry Bridges reminded us, "God has not called us to be like those around us, He has called us to be like Himself. Holiness is nothing less than conformity to the character of God."[56] We are to be in the world, not of the world. Enough with compromising and giving in because it's easier. It is time for God's people to take a stand. We should be setting the example.

Like Daniel and his friends.

Remember them from the last chapter, they decided to obey God's dietary laws rather than defile themselves by trying to fit in with the Babylonian culture (Daniel 1:8). The ones who ate only fruits and vegetables and drank only water were healthier than all of the other young people who were eating from the king's table.

Okay, so we all know that pizza and doughnuts are bad for us, just like we know that fresh veggies and fruit are good for us. Knowing isn't the problem. Doing what's right and sticking to it is another story. Why? Because we are in the habit of eating poorly. Yes, I said *habit*. Our tastes are the result of habits. If you grew up in a different part of the world, in a different culture, you would enjoy different foods. Tastes are created. Therefore, they can be changed. We have to create a new habit of eating healthy.

Speaking of habits, let me share a funny example with you. When our boys, Reese, Sam, and Gabe were about 5, 3 and 1 respectively, I watched them in the mornings while Tracy was at work at St. Jude. I didn't go in to work at the Sheriff's Office until almost 3 p.m., so having opposite shifts was nice. It allowed us to keep our boys at home without having to put them in daycare.

So, I was at home one day fixing the boys some lunch while simultaneously talking on the phone to a customer service rep from AT&T. While I was on hold as she was looking something up, Reese yelled out, "Dad, you forgot my broccoli!" as only a five-year old can. The woman on the phone heard that and couldn't resist.

"Sir," she asked. "Did I just hear a child ask for broccoli?"

Yes, ma'am. That's my son, Reese.

"How old is Reese?" she asked.

He's five.

"How on earth did you get your five-year-old to like broccoli?" she asked almost incredulously.

It's easy, I said, *it's what he knows.*

Parents, if your kids don't like vegetables, may I suggest that it's probably because you aren't feeding them vegetables. Or maybe you could try preparing them a different way. As I said earlier, I don't like mushy broccoli either. I like it nice and crisp and still crunchy. That's how my kids like it too. They love stir-fry veggies!

My point is, start eating healthy as a family. If your kids resist, they will eventually give in. I promise. They won't starve. One of my favorite sayings is, "There are two options at every meal: take it or leave it." As it should be.

One more thing: Since this is a lifestyle, it has to be doable. For starters, it is important to be realistic. Vowing to never eat dessert again as long as you live is unrealistic and will set you up for failure. Not only is this an almost impossible goal, but it's also undesirable.

That's not what I am saying you should do.

Every once in a while I'll enjoy a piece of pie or a really good hamburger and fries. I will usually make them myself with natural ingredients. And, for the record, they taste better—just ask anyone who has had my key lime pie. Conversely, if you allow yourself too much wiggle room, you will find success elusive as well. For example, you may tell yourself that the occasional cheeseburger won't kill you. That's true to a point. It depends on your definition of "occasional." A good general plan is to use the 80/20 rule. If you eat clean 80 percent of the time, you can afford to cheat 20 percent of the time.

Personally, I tend to lean toward 90/10. Part of that is because the longer you eat clean, the less you want to cheat. It's not that you're afraid of gaining a pound or two. It's because you know that you won't feel very good after your indulgence—because you are committed to being fully alive.

CHAPTER 9

THE PILLAR OF FITNESS

In today's technology-driven, plasma-screened-in world, it's easy to forget that we are born movers.[1]
— JOHN J. RATEY, M.D.

Low fitness stood out by far as the single strongest predictor of death— more powerful even than obesity, diabetes, high cholesterol, high blood pressure, and smoking.[2]
— JORDAN METZL, M.D.

All parts of the body which have a function, if used in moderation and exercised in labors in which each is accustomed, become thereby healthy, well developed and age more slowly, but if unused they become liable to disease, defective in growth and age quickly.[3]
— HIPPOCRATES, the father of medicine

Mike was 41 years old when I first met him and his wife, Michelle, in 2009. He was one of the elders at TLC Church and has as much of a servant's heart as anybody I have ever met. So, of course, when Dana asked me to teach on biblical health on Wednesday nights, Mike and Michelle were there. During those six weeks God started working on Mike's heart, telling him that he needed to start taking better care of his health. Mike came to me and asked if I would help him.

It wasn't that Mike was terribly overweight. He only needed to lose about 30 pounds; but he knew he wasn't at his best, and he wasn't happy. He was suffering from depression and was on 100mg of Zoloft (sertraline). He didn't like some of the side effects he was experiencing and wanted off. He knew he could do better—feel better.

Mike decided to start with the exact same program I started with He and Michelle were going to do it together. Besides, he said, "If it worked for you, I knew it could work for me." There is a lot of truth in that. When you have seen someone else have results with something, it gives you hope that you can do it.

But the important thing is not the program he used. It's that Mike got moving. Over the next few months, Mike dropped from 187 pounds to 155 pounds. More important, after just a couple of weeks of working out, Mike started feeling better. He was happier. He had more confidence; and, with his doctor's permission, he stopped taking his Zoloft.

He hasn't needed it since.

Mike and I were talking the other day about his transformation, and it was a great time of reconnecting. We hadn't really talked since my family had moved to Texas a couple of years ago. Mike told me, "I don't know if I could have done it without you. It helps to have a coach helping you out and encouraging you. It helps to have a friend."

It was a little emotional for both of us. I always get emotional when I talk with people whose lives have been dramatically improved through fitness. But he also talked about how many areas of his life improved when he improved his fitness. He said his walk with God was better because the discipline of fitness spilled over into his other spiritual disciplines. Mike and Michelle's marriage also improved.

As Mike said, "When you're fit, you communicate better. You feel like going out more. Your mood improves and that helps everything. You have more confidence. All of those things make for a better marriage."

Yes, they do.

"And you know what else is really fun?" Mike said, "When you can wear your son's clothes."

We both had a good laugh about that one. Now, Mike is about to be a granddad. His son, Justin, and daughter-in-law, Rachel, are expecting their first child in a few months. Mike talked about how active his father-in-law was his whole life and how much he was able to do with Justin when he was growing up. He would do things like taking Justin out riding 4-wheelers on the farm. In contrast, his own father was inactive and didn't get to do as much as he would have liked to with Justin.

"I don't want to be like that with my grandchildren," he said. "I want to be able to play with them and roll around on the floor with them and be there for them as they grow up."

There it is. That's being fully alive for your whole life.

I should probably point out that although this chapter focuses on the exercise component of fitness, optimal fitness is not possible without proper nutrition. You may look good, but you won't be fully alive. I hear people say all the time that the reason they workout is so they can eat whatever they want. That's a lie; and sooner or later, you'll pay for it.

There's a saying, "You can't out-train a bad diet." It's true. But you also can't be at your best without being physically fit because we were made to move.

MADE TO MOVE

It was David, the shepherd, warrior, king and poet, who praised God because He was "fearfully and wonderfully made" (Psalm 139:14). The human body, with all its interconnected and interdependent systems, is an absolute marvel of biomechanical engineering. It is designed for action. We are made to move. Movement makes us happy. Movement makes us healthier. Sitting or lying around watching the world pass us by makes us depressed and sick.

If you are sick and tired of being sick and tired, you have got to get moving.

When God created Adam and placed him in the garden, He put him to work (Genesis 2:15). God created man to be strong as a worker and a warrior. All of us yearn in the deepest places of our hearts for an adventure to share. That includes the ladies. Eve was created as Adam's helper.

Wait, that's not quite right. So much gets lost in translation from the original Hebrew.

When God saw that it was not good for man to be alone, He decided to create Eve. He refers to her as Adam's *ezer kenegdo* (Genesis 2:18). According to the Theological Wordbook of the Old Testament (TWOT), "this word is generally used to designate divine aid."[4] I love the insight on this in John & Stasi Eldredge's *Captivating*. They point out that the word *ezer* is only used 20 other times in the entire Old Testament and "Most of the contexts are life and death . . . and God is your only hope. . . . A better translation therefore of *ezer* would be "lifesaver."[5] *Kenegdo* is a Hebrew preposition that means "in front of" or "corresponding to" and combined with *ezer* here means, "a help corresponding to him i.e. equal and adequate to himself."[6] So, Eve was a strong and vitally important counterpart.

Eve was created to live and work and fight alongside her husband. She was every bit his equal, and she was created to be a source of strength and life. As Eldredge observed, "You don't need a lifesaver if your mission is to be a couch potato. You need an *ezer* when your life is in constant danger. … Eve is essential. She has an irreplaceable role to play. All that human beings were intended to do here on earth—all the creativity and exploration, all the battle and rescue and nurture—we were intended to do *together*."[7]

To do any of those things, we need a certain level of fitness. I'm not saying you need to become an elite athlete, although that certainly doesn't hurt. But you *do* need to be fit enough to perform the functions you were created to accomplish.

Stop it! I saw you cringe. You're thinking, *Great! Now he's going to tell me that I have to start exercising.* No, I'm not. You don't *have* to. But I *am* going to show you why you should *want* to start exercising.

Over the past few years, we have been seeing an increasing awareness of the need for physical fitness in the body of Christ. Still, some folks remain resistant, claiming that physical fitness is a waste of time or even sinful. To support their view, they quote the Apostle Paul in 1 Timothy 1:8: "For while bodily training is of some value, godliness is of value in every way, as it holds promise for the present life and also for the life to come" (1 Timothy 4:8 ESV).

By this point it should be abundantly clear from Scripture that God is concerned about what we do with and how we care for our physical bodies, so how are we to interpret this verse? For years I have heard people erroneously take Paul's emphasis on godliness over physical training to mean that physical exercise is of *no* value. They imply that investing time for exercise is "worldly" and somehow interferes with godliness. But that is *not* what Paul is saying. In fact, we have already established from Scripture that God is greatly concerned about our bodies. We also have to consider the context of the passage itself.

Albert Barnes commented, "The apostle does not mean to say that bodily exercise is in itself unproper, or that no advantage can be derived from it in the preservation of health; but he refers to it solely as a means of religion; as supposed to promote holiness of heart and of life."[8]

Colossians 2:23 is widely regarded as a parallel text to 1 Timothy 4:8. There, Paul said, "These have indeed an appearance of wisdom in promoting self-made religion and asceticism and severity to the body, but they are of no value in stopping the indulgence of the flesh" (Colossians 2:23 ESV). In this case, Paul was referring to extreme asceticism as a man-made religion—which runs contrary to the work of Christ.

Ascetics neglected the body by putting on sackcloth and ashes. They subjected themselves to extreme testings and painful penances. Their appearance became like that of a slave beaten and living in absolute poverty. These might seem like acts of humility and piety, but they were really motivated by pride and selfishness. This is the exact opposite of what we are talking about. They actually took great pride in how much they neglected the body as if it had no value, when we know that God created the body as well as the soul—and that He cares for both.

Paul said bodily exercise is of some value but godliness is more valuable. Amen. But God is not confined to one area of our lives—He is Lord of all. Godliness includes fitness. It was also Paul who said, "I discipline my body and keep it under control" (1 Corinthians 9:27 ESV). As we saw earlier how 1 Corinthians 9:25-27 holds athletes up as an example of how we should pursue godliness. We discipline our bodies, not as a form of religion or to gain God's favor, but out of love and devotion for the One who created us. It's a sincere desire to offer to Him our best.

Paul instructed Timothy to reject false teaching, which is harmful to us spiritually, and to exercise ourselves toward godliness. He then reaffirmed the benefit of physical exercise to use it as an example of the greater benefit of spiritual exercise. Bodily exercise, while beneficial in this life will not result in eternal life; nevertheless, Paul very clearly said that physical exercise does benefit. I am reminded of Jesus' instruction to the Pharisees: "What sorrow awaits you teachers of religious law and you Pharisees. Hypocrites! For you are careful to tithe even the tiniest income from your herb gardens, but you ignore the more important aspects of the law— justice, mercy, and faith. You should tithe, yes, but do not neglect the more important things." (Matthew 23:23 NLT)

It is not a case of "either/or" but of "both/and." We need to exercise ourselves bodily and spiritually. To assume that Paul was teaching Timothy that Christians should not engage in physical exercise is to fall into the Gnostic heresy of separating physical from spiritual. And that ignores the whole of Scripture's teaching about how we care for and offer our bodies to God.

Another fundamental rule of interpreting Scripture is that you have to consider the original audience along with the distance of time. Paul wrote these words to Timothy nearly two thousand years ago. They lived in a time and culture where constant physical activity was the norm. It has only been within the last 150 years that labor-saving devices have produced a drastic decline of our daily physical activity. In 2004, a study entitled *Physical Activity in an Old Order Amish Community* demonstrated that the Amish, who reject modern conveniences, had a very high level of activity integrated into their daily lives.[9]

"The Amish were able to show us just how far we've fallen in the last 150 years or so in terms of the amount of physical activity we typically perform," said David R. Bassett, Ph.D., FACSM, a professor at the University of Tennessee, Knoxville, and lead researcher for the study. "Their lifestyle indicates that physical activity played a critical role in keeping our ancestors fit and healthy."[10]

On average, the Amish participated in six times the physical activity performed by participants in a recent survey of 12 modernized nations. That's "almost mind boggling," says Bassett. "If somebody runs 10 to 15 miles a day, I think that's probably the same level of [energy] expenditure as the Amish farmer."[11]

Are you beginning to see what's going on here? Paul was advocating the benefits of physical exercise in a culture that was much more active than we are. How much more important it is for us to engage in physical exercise! Dr. John J. Ratey, clinical associate professor of psychiatry at Harvard Medical School commented:

> In today's technology-driven, plasma-screened-in world, it's easy to forget that we are born movers . . . because we've engineered movement right out of our lives. . . The sedentary character of modern life is a disruption of our nature and it poses one of the biggest threats to our continued survival. . . . we're literally killing ourselves.[12]

Dr. Ted Mitchell, the president and medical director of the world-renowned Cooper Clinic in Texas stated:

> We know unequivocally, beyond any shadow of a doubt, that a sedentary lifestyle directly causes chronic disease and a shorter life span regardless of whether you are thin, overweight or obese. . . Twice as many people die from sedentary living than from viruses and bacteria, and more die from inactivity than from firearms, illicit use of drugs, sexually transmitted diseases, and automobile accidents combined.[13]

A couple of years ago, Dr. Steven Blair from the University of South Carolina's Arnold School for Public Health quantified the effects of various health risks on the likelihood of dying for a group of 50,000 men and women. Blair calculated how much less likely it was for a person to die if he or she eliminated certain risk factors: if a smoker kicked the habit, for example, or if an obese person lost the extra baggage.

> Low fitness stood out by far as the single strongest predictor of death—more powerful even than obesity, diabetes, high cholesterol, high blood pressure, and smoking. With the exception of high blood

pressure, which ran a close second, compared to the risks associated with being unfit, the other factors were small potatoes. It wasn't even close. In fact, the research shows that if you're highly fit when in your eighties, you're less likely to die than if you're unfit when in your sixties.[14]

Remember, this is not just about being thin. We learned that it's common for people who control their weight through diet alone to have large fat deposits around their interior organs called visceral fat. Over the last few years, research has uncovered a striking correlation between visceral fat and two major health issues: heart disease and type 2 diabetes. This interior fat is extremely responsive to physical activity. Optimal health is only achieved through both diet and exercise.

A 2004 article in the New England Journal of Medicine concluded that liposuction of surface fat does not affect your cholesterol or blood sugar, demonstrating that this layer of fat is not physiologically important. The answer to visceral fat is not liposuction. It's behavior, and specifically, physical activity.[15]

WHY YOU WANT TO EXERCISE

Ok, enough with the facts for now. I promised I would help you discover why you want to exercise. Are you ready? I'll begin by letting my friend and mentor, Denise Needham, share her story:

Growing up in the Midwest, my family was not focused on fitness as an important part of your health. We ate mostly from the farm and gardens, which was good; but other than the occasional days my mother would work out to Jack LaLanne, the training just wasn't there. What I did notice about my body, is I loved sports. I enjoyed diving into the pool and competing. Playing softball in junior high and being on the swim team in high school all felt natural and necessary for me to keep up with the stresses of school and striving for straight "A's." When I was married and after delivering my son, I had gained more than 50 pounds during that pregnancy. I couldn't wait to take the extra weight off so I began jogging and dieting. Even after the birth of my daughter, which also had a 50-pound weight gain, I purchased an exercise bike due to the long cold winters in Nebraska. I wanted to exercise and get back to my high school weight and size. I also found that my mood and emotions shifted when I was regularly exercising. Where it was easy to get depressed with the cabin fever of the winter season, working out changed all that. And, frankly, I became addicted to exercising everyday no matter what.

Throughout the years there have been the up's and downs of life where I have gone back and forth from a sedentary lifestyle to training to run a marathon. In training, I felt invincible; and this euphoric strength impacted how well I performed in my career. They seemed to go hand in hand. Even to this day, now that I am in my 60s, my body, mind and soul have learned through repeated recoveries that turning my back on exercise comes at a dear cost. Weight gain, depression, digestive issues, and the list goes on and on as my health spirals downward. But once I get back up on the bike, in the pool or on the trails, it all turns around again. I know it's because that's how God made me, and now I also want to continue to maintain a vibrant lifestyle. I fight the good fight of faith to stay active again, "no matter what" and now to glorify Christ in my life.

Now it's your turn. Before I begin working with a new client, I have them fill out a health survey. That's because before you begin any new journey you have to have a clear picture of your starting point. So, let's get started: Do you like what you see when you look in a mirror? Be honest, but don't be critical.

How would you describe your current fitness level? How do you feel about it? What do you notice about your face? What do you notice about your neck, shoulders, chest, arms, abs, legs and glutes? How are your energy levels? Do you have tons of energy or do you find yourself surviving on caffeine and energy drinks? Do you have any concerns when it comes to your health? Do you have a family history of heart disease or diabetes or cancer?

Now that you have taken a good overall assessment of your health, here is the kicker: How is your current fitness level impacting other areas of your life—your family, your relationships, your faith, your ability to engage in ministry opportunities, your ability to play with your kids or grandkids, your self-esteem, your focus, your ability to think clearly, your ability to make good decisions, healthy decisions? Am I missing anything? You see, your fitness affects far more than just your body—it affects every area of your life.

The next step is to paint a new picture. I tell my prospective clients to paint a detailed picture of their future selves—maybe a year into the future. Then two years. Then five years. Go ahead and stretch it to 20 years.

Picture in your mind you at your ideal fitness level. Forget about what you think you can do. What do you want?

Picture yourself *Fully Alive!* You are living and enjoying life at every level—physically, mentally, spiritually, relationally. What do you see? How do you feel? How's your confidence? Your productivity? Your sex life? Got it?

What can you do then that you can't do now? How is your life different? What do you enjoy? Now you're creating a movie in your mind. You see the life you were intended to live—life at its fullest.

Now, just to make sure this sinks in, we have to do the opposite. Picture yourself in the future, maybe five or 10 or 20 years down the road—only this time you haven't made any changes. You still eat the same way. Maybe you made a few changes, but nothing too severe. You still aren't finding time to exercise. If you've been gaining an average of five pounds a year, which is fairly average, you're 10 pounds heavier in just two years and 100 pounds heavier in 20 years. How does that sound? Even if you only gain two pounds a year, it's still 10 extra pounds in five years and 40 in 20 years. Not the direction you want to be going.

What about your energy levels? How do you feel? What sort of mood are you in? How's your confidence now? Your productivity? Are you fully alive or struggling to even survive?

Now choose. Everything in life that has value is hard. That's the way it is. But you know what, taking the easy way is actually harder in the long run. It's the narrow road that leads to life. The easy way leads to destruction. Which way will you go? Which life do you choose? Because the decisions you make right now determine which life you will end up with.

Have you decided? Great! Let's get moving.

MOVEMENT IS MEDICINE

Hippocrates was right. Movement is medicine just like food is. Combined, they are exponentially more powerful. Regular exercise helps us to fight off disease and the effects of aging. And it helps us live longer. In his book, *The Exercise Cure: A Doctor's All-Natural, No-Pill Prescription for Better Health and Longer Life,* Dr. Jordan Metzl, stated unequivocally, "The miracle medicine that works across every disease state is called exercise. . . . Science has shown again and again, across all manner of diseases, maladies, and health risks, that exercise can prevent, improve, or outright cure your symptoms."[16]

The good news is that you can start reaping the benefits of being more active from the moment you begin. Exercise is medicine. Dr. Metzl went on to say:

Exercise is honest, inexpensive, all-natural medicine. It's also the easiest, cheapest, and fastest way to a happy life. When formerly sedentary people start moving regularly, miraculous things happen— just as miraculous as any treatment or procedure or drug I've ever seen or prescribed in my medical career.[17]

As a former couch potato, I can attest to the incredible benefits of physical activity. You've got to move it, or you will lose it—your health, your functionality, your physique, your freedom, your ability to fully enjoy life—your life itself. Dr. Daniel Amen said, "Physical exercise is the fountain of youth; it's critical to keeping your brain vibrant and young. If you want to attack Alzheimer's, depression, obesity, and aging all at once, move every day."[18]

The purpose of this chapter is to touch lightly on some of the primary scientifically-proven benefits of exercise. We don't have nearly enough room in this book to go into all of the miraculous benefits of exercise— entire books are devoted to the subject and most of them still just scratch the surface. I'll try to hit the highlights of the "big ones" and then list a few others for you. The research is out there. If you want to learn more, you can find plenty of resources.

Maybe in the future I'll write another book just on this one topic.

MOVE FOR YOUR MIND

The first benefit of exercise may surprise you—I know it did me at first. We need to move for *our mind*. Yes, you heard right, exercise is good for your brain. In the introduction of his book *Spark: The Revolutionary New Science of Exercise and the Brain*, Dr. John J. Ratey said:

We all know that exercise makes us feel better, but most of us have no idea why. We assume it's because we're burning off stress or reducing muscle tension or boosting endorphins, and we leave it at that. But the real reason we feel so good when we get our blood pumping is that it makes the brain function at its best, and in my view, this benefit of physical activity is far more important—and fascinating—than what it does for the body. Building muscles and conditioning the heart and lungs are essentially side effects. I often tell my patients that the point of exercise is to build and condition the brain.[19]

You're waiting for the catch, right? Well, you're right. There has to be some drawback to exercise. But the catch isn't really with exercise; it's with our attitudes. For exercise to reach its full potential in our lives, it has to be voluntary—forced workouts don't quite seem to do the trick. No worries though, as long as you get to the point where you want to exercise, you have the ability to change your future—not just physically but mentally.

Dr. Carl Cotman, director of the Institute of Brain Aging and Dementia at the University of California, Irvine, found a link between physical activity and mental ability. Cotman's study found that a compound called BDNF (Brain-Derived Neurotropic Factor) is increased with exercise. BDNF, says Ratey "improves the function of neurons, encourages their growth, and strengthens and protects them against the natural process of cell death. And . . . BDNF is a crucial biological link between thought, emotions, and movement."[20] He calls it "Miracle-Grow for the brain."[21]

Not only does exercise stimulate the creation of new brain cells (neurons), but it also strengthens the connection between those cells. The areas of the brain that are stimulated through exercise are associated with memory and learning. Cotman said, "One of the prominent features of exercise, which is sometimes not appreciated in studies, is an improvement in the rate of learning, and I think that's a really cool take-home message because it suggests that if you're in good shape, you may be able to learn and function more efficiently."[22]

According to Ratey research shows "physical activity sparks biological changes that encourage brain cells to bind to one another. For the brain to learn, these connections must be made. . . . The more neuroscientists discover about this process, the clearer it becomes that exercise provides an unparalleled stimulus, creating an environment in which the brain is ready, willing, and able to learn."[23]

Moving the body keeps the brain functioning and growing. And that's a good thing. Because as Ratey said, "If your brain isn't actively growing, then it's dying."[24]

This is extremely important as we get older. Exercise is critical for maintaining mental clarity and focus, as well as keeping the brain sharp as we age. That's a pretty cool bonus no matter how old you are. It is even believed that activity can help prevent Alzheimer's disease, dementia, and other mental disorders that are generally associated with aging.

I hate when I hear people talk about the "normal" effects of aging. Losing mental function is not the "normal" result of aging. It's what we have come to accept as normal. My maternal grandfather, I called him

"Da-Daw," was sharp as a tack right up until the day he died, and he was active his whole life.

Henriette Van Praag, a staff scientist at the Salk Institute for Biological Studies, says, "I would absolutely recommend people exercise for the mental benefits—especially the elderly. People don't care about whether they're a size four or a six as they get older. But they do care where their car keys are and whether they'll have the ability to play card games and enjoy life."[25]

So much for the excuse, "I'm too old to workout." Nonsense. The older you are, the more important it is for you to exercise—if for no other reason than the mental benefits.

Oh, and here's another bonus! Exercise does something that until recently the experts said was impossible—it encourages the growth of *new* brain cells through a process called neurogenesis. "For the better part of the twentieth century, scientific dogma held that the brain was hardwired once fully developed in adolescence, meaning we're born with all the neurons we're going to get. . . . But guess what? They do grow back—by the thousands."[26] That's right, you can actually grow new brain cells, and exercise plays a crucial role. Ratey said, "What I find interesting, though, is that relatively few scientists are studying exercise because they're interested in exercise. Rather, they make the mice run because it 'massively increases neurogenesis.'"[27] They do this so they can deconstruct the chain of signals behind the process of neurogenesis. In Ratey's words, "That's what the pharmaceutical companies need to create drugs. They dream of an anti-Alzheimer's pill that regenerates neurons to keep memory intact. ... Just imagine if they could put exercise in a bottle."[28] So if you feel like you're losing your mind, you don't need a pill, there's not one—you just need to exercise more.

But wait, there's more. If you are studying for a test, you're better off getting up and getting a quick workout in than just sitting there studying. A German study conducted in 2007 showed that people learn vocabulary words 20 percent faster after exercise than before exercise—and that the rate of learning correlated directly with levels of BDNF in the brain.[29] Who knew? Well, obviously God knew.

Bottom line? In Ratey's words: "Exercise is the single most powerful tool you have to optimize your brain function."[30]

MOVE TO REDUCE STRESS

Feeling stressed out? Start moving, and you will start to feel better—almost immediately. Numerous studies have shown that one of the best ways to reduce stress is through exercise. When we are stressed, our bodies release a chain-reaction of chemicals as part of the "fight or flight" response. If you are in a situation where you need to run away from something or stand and fight a threat, the stress response is helpful. It is a means of survival.

In today's society, we don't have to fight for our lives most of the time; and we lead sedentary lives, so we don't really have a way to burn off the stress or pent-up negative emotions. As a result, the stress chemicals stay in our body creating emotional and physical problems. Exercise can help by providing an outlet for negative emotions such as worry, irritability, depression, hostility, anger, frustration, and anxiety. Regular exercise is the best way to manage the fight or flight response, and it helps our bodies return to a balanced state more quickly.

MOVE AGAINST DEPRESSION

Depression hits for a number of reasons, and often the external cause is clear. Major life events such as the death of a loved one, a divorce, the loss of a job, or moving can trigger depression. It also can be hormonal. For women, depression may be a symptom of menopause. For men, it could be a drop in testosterone. Thyroid problems can cause depression. So can lack of sleep. Some pharmaceuticals are known to cause depression. (Just watch the commercials and see how many of them list depression as a side effect. Even the depression medications list suicidal tendencies as a possible side effect.)

Depression can also be spiritual in nature—whether we are under attack or just feel separated from God.

Whatever the cause, exercise is known to be nature's antidepressant, and plenty of studies prove that. In September of 2000 researchers from Duke University made worldwide news with a study showing that exercise is as effective as sertraline (Zoloft) at treating depression long-term.

> After demonstrating that 30 minutes of brisk exercise three times a week is just as effective as drug therapy in relieving the symptoms of major depression in the short term, medical center researchers have now shown that continued exercise greatly reduces the chances of the depression returning. . . . The new study, which followed the same participants for an additional six months, found that patients who continued to exercise after completing the initial trial were much less likely to see their depression return than the other patients. Only 8 percent of patients in the exercise group had their

depression return, while 38 percent of the drug-only group and 31 percent of the exercise-plus-drug group relapsed.[31]

Did you catch that last part? The exercise only group relapsed at nearly a quarter the rate of the exercise-plus-medication group. Exercise worked better long term than the combination of exercise and medication. What great news! So why haven't we heard more about this? Unfortunately, the story got buried. When the *New York Times* ran the story in October of 2000, it was tucked back on page 14 of the "Health and Fitness" section. News like this rarely finds its way to the headlines, it tends to get buried. Do you ever wonder why that is? I do. Ratey is right, "If exercise came in pill form, it would be plastered across the front page, hailed as the blockbuster drug of the century."[32]

Dr. Mitchell explained it like this: "Treating depression with medication, while necessary in many cases, is also a double-edged sword. You alleviate the symptoms temporarily, but side effects can be substantial and the pills are expensive. People tend to not stay on the program and to stop taking medication within six months. Physical activity, on the other hand, makes you feel better, healthier, and happier."[33]

April had always been thin growing up, but after the birth of her first child she began to struggle with her weight for the first time in her life. She tried this diet and that diet; and for years, she did the whole yo-yo of losing weight and gaining it back. The pounds she lost always seemed to come back and bring friends with them. She had also battled eating disorders and extreme social anxiety for years. When we first met at a park where both of our children played, she was 33, had three wonderful kids, and a thriving business. But her weight had ballooned above 200 pounds, and her health was nowhere near where she needed it to be. She could barely walk from her car into the mall if she couldn't find a close parking space. Climbing stairs became a herculean task, and she would get so out of breath that she had to take breaks. She knew it was time. She knew she needed to do something.

When April first began working with me, she admitted it was a real challenge at first. In her words:

I pretty much gave up before I ever got started. I just was not completely committed. I gave up quickly and then gained more weight. From two steps behind square one—but ready to make some real changes—I began again!! But this time my heart was devoted and I knew that I had to do this for me and for my family.

The challenge in front of me was great, and sometimes seemed impossible, but I pressed on and pushed through it. Truly, the only reason I had the will to try is because I had seen some amazing success stories from people at all different weights and stages of life. I saw their ups and downs and accepted them from the beginning. I dove in head first with no reservations. No more excuses or pity parties. No more hiding the numbers on the scales from everyone. Setting my pride aside, I began for really the first time to take care of me and get healthy!

I rejected failure—for the first time. I said, I *will* do this! It takes that mental connection to do this, otherwise the success will not come. You must embrace the journey on all levels—the good and the bad—and tackle it! It can be done! The sky is the limit!"

April ended up losing nearly 80 pounds! She said:

This has changed me forever and I feel like I am really living. No more being afraid to leave the house. No more looking down so that nobody looks at me as I walk into a room. No more hiding behind people. This feels really good, and the journey is just amazing. The old April never would have believed that she could accomplish so much; but once I decided to go for it with all of my heart and soul, nothing could stand in my way. Each and every workout was full of my heart.

I cannot imagine my life ever being any different again. I live a very full life and get to enjoy so much now that I never could before. If I am ever having a hard day, my workouts are where I find my center, and I can find that mountaintop again.

MOVE TO STOP METABOLIC SYNDROME

What's metabolic syndrome? If that's your question, I understand. I didn't know either until I found out that I had it in 2006.

It's really a combination of things. If you find yourself complaining a lot about low energy levels or general disease, this may be the culprit. Metabolic syndrome significantly increases your risk of obesity, killer diseases (such as heart disease, diabetes, and cancer), physical frailty, and premature death. If you have three or more of the following five characteristics, you are at very high risk—with four times the chance of developing coronary heart disease and three times the chance of developing diabetes.

Those risk factors include the following:

- Your waist circumference is greater than 35 inches for a woman or greater than 40 inches for a man.
- Your fasting blood sugar is above 100 mg/dl
- Your triglycerides (blood fats) are more than 150 mg/dl
- Your HDL is less than 50 mg/dl for a woman and less than 40 mg/dl for a man
- Your blood pressure is higher than 130/85—or you need to take a blood pressure medication.[34]

According to Dr. Mitchell, "this collection of risk factors could very well be called 'the physical inactivity syndrome.' That's because a sedentary lifestyle contributes directly to each and every element in the cluster."[35]

Even though metabolic syndrome is recognized as an epidemic by medical researchers and public health agencies, it also hasn't received a lot of attention. That's because it sort of sneaks up on you—it's a silent killer. Dr. Mitchell says, "Patients typically aren't sick or ailing, even if they have several or more of the risk factors. They don't have hypertension, even if their blood pressure is slightly high. They don't have diabetes, even though their blood sugar is slightly high. And they don't have high cholesterol. Usually they have what we call 'watch and wait' values for blood pressure, blood sugar, and cholesterol. They don't know they are already at risk. Right out of the blue they could have a heart attack."[36]

In addition, no medications are designed to treat this collection of risk factors, so the pharmaceutical industry isn't bombarding you with ads promoting their miracle "breakthrough" cure. Honestly, they have no answer for this one. They can't put exercise in pill form.

No worries though, because there is a cure: All you need to do is get moving. Metabolic syndrome is directly linked to a sedentary lifestyle, and exercise is effective at preventing and reversing all of the risk factors.

A bulging waistline, even if you're otherwise thin, means that you are carrying large deposits of visceral fat around your organs. Visceral fat is different from the subcutaneous fat that is just under your skin—and it's much more dangerous. This fat is directly linked to a sedentary lifestyle, and people who maintain their weight through diet alone rather than exercise are still likely to have large deposits of this internal fat. This is commonly viewed as the number one risk factor for metabolic syndrome.[37] The good news is that visceral fat is extremely reactive to physical activity, so even a little bit of exercise can go a long way.

Elevated blood sugar indicates that your body is not processing glucose effectively, but you have not yet progressed to the point of diabetes. The good thing is that this too is easily regulated by exercise, and the effects begin immediately. Glucose (sugar) is stored in muscle tissue and serves as the primary source of fuel for your muscles. Even a small amount of exercise increases your body's ability to burn sugar and will begin to normalize levels of glucose in your blood.

This effect is immediate and continues for up to 48 hours, especially if you have higher blood sugar levels. Since working out and using your muscles improves blood sugar, regular exercise helps prevent metabolic syndrome and prevents it from progressing to full blown diabetes.

It's also no secret that physical activity has a powerful positive impact on both cholesterol and triglycerides. There is good cholesterol (HDL) and bad cholesterol (LDL). HDL protects against heart disease; and while a few medications claim to increase HDL levels, none of them are very good at it. And all of those come with negative side effects. Exercise, however, is extremely effective has only good side effects, especially combined with a healthy diet. Physical activity also lowers triglyceride levels relatively quickly.

And if you have elevated blood pressure, exercise is widely recognized to lower blood pressure in nearly every case. In fact, one session of physical activity can help normalize blood pressure for up to forty-eight hours. Dr. Mitchell said, "Our work at the center shows that physical activity substantially lowers the risk of dying prematurely even for individuals with resistant high blood pressure."[38] Translation: Even when nothing else seems to control your blood pressure, exercise significantly lowers your risk of dying from it.

MOVE AGAINST CARDIOVASCULAR DISEASE

Cardiovascular disease will kill more than 600,000 Americans this year. We have already seen it referred to as a completely preventable foodborne illness, but it is also highly responsive to exercise. According to Dr. Mitchell, "Our research and experience with patients tell us without a doubt one of the most important things—perhaps the most important thing—you can do to prevent a heart attack or stroke is to be physically active. And for patients who already have the disease, it reduces complications."[39]

Several studies support this position, most notably the Framingham Heart Study, which definitively showed that "regular, longterm physical exertion protects against death from cardiovascular disease."[40] The

Framingham study began in 1948 with more than 5,200 people whom researchers followed for decades. Then, in 1971, 5,100 of their children were signed on and followed. In 2002, a third generation was added to the study, and it continues on to this day. I'd say that's a pretty comprehensive and authoritative study, wouldn't you? And the results have been verified by numerous other studies from all around the world.

If heart disease is a completely foodborne illness and regular exercise protects against death from heart disease, imagine if you combined exercise and a healthy diet. The cure for heart disease is already here. If everyone started doing these things, it is conceivable that we could almost completely eradicate heart disease within just a few years. Of course, not everyone will. Will you?

MOVE AGAINST DIABETES

The Diabetes Prevention Program conducted a study that demonstrated how simple lifestyle changes prevent or delay Type 2 diabetes across ethnic and cultural lines. Exercise is an important part of this. As we have already seen, exercise has a tremendous effect on blood sugar and helps to regulate blood glucose levels. If you have been completely sedentary, your first step may be just that—start walking. You can start with just 30-minutes a day three or four days a week. As your fitness level improves, increase the intensity of your workouts.

Several studies suggest that people with diabetes and pre-diabetes can get even greater benefits from more intense forms of exercise, such as high intensity interval training (HIIT). A 2007 study published in the Annals of Internal Medicine showed that an exercise program combining both strength training and aerobic training is more effective at controlling blood sugar than either one by itself.

MOVE AGAINST CANCER

Research gives us a lot of evidence that demonstrates the importance and effectiveness of exercise in preventing several common forms of cancer, most notably colon and breast cancer.

According to Dr. Metzl, "A 2008 research review found that, across the board, exercise may increase survival rates following a cancer diagnosis by up to 60 percent. A second study found that, in women recovering from breast cancer treatment, a combined program of aerobic and resistance training produced "large and rapid improvements in health-related outcomes." A third study, this one from 2012, found that people with advanced-stage cancer who exercised had lower levels of psychological anxiety, stress, and depression, and improved levels of physical pain, fatigue, shortness of breath, constipation, and insomnia."[41]

Dr. I-Min Lee, assistant professor of medicine at Harvard University, is an expert on the relationship between physical activity and life-expectancy. She has done intensive studies on the effect of exercise on non-communicable diseases, including cancer. Dr. Lee gathered and analyzed the data from studies published in various medical journals and discovered the following links between physical activity and cancer prevention:

- Active individuals had a 30-40 percent reduction in the risk of developing colon cancer compared to inactive people
- Physically active women had about a 20-30 percent reduced risk of breast cancer.
- Individuals who were physically active had a lower risk of lung cancer.[42]

In 1996, James Kampert, a veteran researcher at the Cooper Clinic studied the relationship between physical activity and cancer mortality alone. His study included more than 25,000 men and 7,000 women who had been examined at the Cooper Clinic prior to 1989. The data showed that those who were physically active had a much lower risk of dying from cancer than those who were not active. This puzzled the experts, so they began looking for possible connections.[43]

Mitchell said, "One theory is that regular physical activity increases the blood flow of natural killer (NK) cells, specific types of white blood cells. Rather than targeting bacteria, viruses, or fungi, they search out cells that look abnormal, such as cancer cells. They search and destroy, and cleanse the body. By increasing the circulation of NK cells, you likely improve your body's detection and destruction of cancer cells."[44]

We also know that recent studies suggest that regular physical activity reduces certain inflammatory molecules in the body that are suspected in the development of certain types of cancer. Plus, physical activity helps a great deal in cancer treatment in the following ways:[45]

- Physical activity may reduce the likelihood of cancer recurrence and enhance survival through its capacity to improve bodily movement, reduce fatigue, and enhance immune function.
- Moderate physical activity reduces relapses and fatigue, while helping patients cope with their illness.

- Physical activity after a breast cancer diagnosis may reduce the risk of death from the disease.

AND THE LIST GOES ON

As I mentioned, entire books have been dedicated to the vast health benefits of exercise. For the sake of space, I will just list a few of the other benefits here. If you would like to learn more about these benefits, I recommend you read *Move Yourself* and *The Exercise Cure*. You can also find much of this online.

- It reduces the risk of stroke
- It helps normalize blood pressure
- It increases bone density and helps prevents osteoporosis
- It improves energy levels
- It improves sleep
- It improves sex
- It improves skin tone
- It reduces pain
- It improves digestion and elimination
- It reduces negative effects of menopause
- It improves confidence levels
- It helps control addictive behavior.

MOVE TO LIVE BETTER, LONGER

The legendary Chuck Norris turned 77 in March 2017. The American martial artist, actor, film producer, screenwriter, and veteran has numerous accomplishments to his name. Since 2005, Norris went viral with the famous "Chuck Norris" memes that had everyone talking and laughing. One of my favorites is, "When the boogeyman goes to sleep at night, he checks his closet for Chuck Norris."

These memes, with their over-the-top hyperbole, make Norris seem invincible and nearly immortal. While he may not be immortal, Norris has certainly aged well, and he credits his longevity to his fitness.

"What I learned long ago is that a physically active lifestyle also improves every aspect of living," he said. "The good news is that you don't have to train like an athlete, you just have to make it a priority."[46]

Not long ago, my oldest son, Reese, and I were watching the TobyMac video for *Till The Day I Die (Live)*. I absolutely love that song! I mentioned that I had gone to the same church as Toby when I lived in Nashville and that, like me, he was also a graduate of Liberty University. Then I mentioned that I started listening to DC Talk (the group he formed with Michael Tait and Kevin Max Smith while they were at Liberty) when I was in college.

"How old is he?" Reese asked.

When I told him Toby was 52, Reese was shocked.

"How can he be so hip?" he asked incredulously.

I just laughed and thought to myself: *Do you see how active he is? That's what this song is about. It's about serving God with everything you have until the day you die. He's all in. The only way he can do that is by staying fit and active, so he does.*

My favorite line in the song—"You say you doin' work, but you're asking where the couch at. How you doin' work when you asking where the couch at?"[47]

It's time to get off the couch. Start by simply moving more. Take the stairs instead of the escalator or elevator. Walk around your house during commercial breaks. Get up from your desk at work from time to time and walk around for a couple of minutes. Just start moving. You will soon find yourself wanting to do more and more as you begin to reap the benefits of movement. We are made to move.

NO PAIN, NO GAIN

You have probably heard the expression, "No Pain, No Gain"—maybe on a shirt proudly worn by someone who obviously works out a lot. It is a saying most often associated with athletics and physical exercise, but its application is universal.

Paul said, "For momentary, light affliction is producing for us an eternal weight of glory far beyond all comparison" (2 Corinthians 4:17 NASB). Paul suffered a lot of persecution. In fact, suffering is a hallmark of the Christian life. Everyone suffers. But whatever we suffer for the sake of the Gospel can't compare to our reward. That "glory" will be infinitely greater than whatever we sacrificed. If you want a closer walk with Jesus, you are going to have to develop the disciplines of reading your Bible and praying every day—for starters.

The author of Hebrews wrote, "Therefore, since we are surrounded by such a great cloud of witnesses, let us throw off everything that hinders and the sin that so easily entangles. And let us run with perseverance the race marked out for us, fixing our eyes on Jesus, the pioneer and perfecter of faith. For the joy set before him he endured the cross, scorning its shame, and sat down at the right hand of the throne of God" (Hebrews 12:1–2 NIV). Lack of fitness hobbles us and slows us down. We are easily entangled by the sins of gluttony and sloth. But Hebrews challenges us to look to Jesus as our example. He endured the horrors of the cross because of His love for us, because what it purchased was worth it to Him.

His sacrifice purchased you, and it purchased me. How can we not lay our own lives and desires down for Him? It doesn't cost us anything close to what it cost Him, yet we are rewarded in both this life and the next. It should be a no-brainer.

Dave Ramsey, author and creator of Financial Peace University, has built an empire teaching people the biblical principles of finances and wealth management. He is always saying, "Live like no one else now so later you can live—and give—like no one else." For 25 years, he's challenged people to stop worrying about what everybody else thinks and to develop the discipline to get on a budget and get out of debt. Do it with the intensity of a gazelle running to escape the cheetah that wants him for dinner.[48]

If you want a thriving, love-filled marriage, it takes work. If you want happy, healthy, well-adjusted kids, it takes work. If you want to advance in your chosen career path, you have to stand out.

And if you want to live better and longer—if you want to be fully alive—it's going to take work.

As I was finishing up a Mixed Martial Arts inspired workout one morning, one of the trainers was telling the other trainer how great she felt. I thought to myself, *I feel great too!*

My oldest son, Reese, was working out with me. When I asked him how he felt, he said "Tired, but good. It feels good."

It does feel good. That's because all those feel-good endorphins flood through your body and brain during exercise. Even on days that I start out not feeling "into it," I always start feeling better within about 15 minutes—and I never, ever regret it.

Which reminds me of a funny texting conversation we had with our friend, Sarah, the other day. She recently found out that she's pregnant—blessing number seven on the way!—and commented that she was laying on the couch trying not to throw up. I love what she said next: "Growing babies—it ain't for the faint-hearted."

I couldn't help but laugh because she's right.

Tracy replied, "No it's not. The first trimester with Reese I didn't think I would ever have another one. Then you get to the end and never want to stop!"

If you've ever been pregnant, you know exactly what she's talking about. If you've ever lived with a woman who is pregnant, you know how crazy it gets. I distinctly remember calling my mom when Tracy was pregnant with Reese. It was toward the end of the first trimester and Tracy had just taken my head off because she could still smell the tuna I had fixed for lunch earlier in the day. I washed the can out and threw it in the trash; but apparently when you're pregnant, you develop a bloodhound's sense of smell. Having never been pregnant, I had no idea.

Anyway, I called my mom and said something along the lines of, *Help! What do I do? She's crazy.* Mom, of course, had the best advice in the world. "Just love her," she said, "She's dealing with a lot and her hormones and body are all out of whack. Just be patient and love her."

Don't you just love the wisdom of moms?

Sarah wrote back to Tracy, "Hahaha right! It's amazing how we forget the bad." It is amazing.

Yeah, I replied. *In the hospital right after Reese was born Tracy said something about that not being so bad and wanting to do it again and I asked her where she had been for the past 9 months.*

We all had a good laugh at that point. Tracy pointed out, "It's the endorphins! If it weren't for the endorphins, I don't think anyone would have more than one!"

Ah, the endorphins. Those same amazing chemicals we get from working out make the whole thing worth it. They help us forget the pain we just went through. And what the temporary pain produces it priceless. We have four amazing children now. Sarah is about to have her seventh. Our friends who have been through the process of adopting a child, tell us how difficult and gut-wrenching it is at times. Parenting is still hard. We still have to work at it, and it never stops; but it is absolutely one of the most rewarding experiences of life.

Developing and maintaining your fitness is no different.

No pain, no gain.

GETTING STARTED

They say it's the start that stops most people. It's one thing to know we should do something and a completely different thing to actually start doing it. Maybe it's uncertainty or not knowing how to start that has been holding you back. I get asked all of the time what the best exercise program is. Easy. It's the one you will actually do.

You might laugh it off, but I'm serious. You might hate working out simply because you haven't found an activity you enjoy yet—or, more likely, you just forgot how much you enjoyed it. I bet if I asked five-year old you if you enjoyed running and playing, you'd smile and scream, "Yes!"

Maybe you prefer working out with weights or cardio or you love dance-based workouts. Maybe you enjoy martial arts. Maybe you like programs like tai chi or yoga. Maybe you're one of those crazy people who enjoys running. Maybe it's rock climbing or skating or biking or basketball or baseball. The options are unlimited. So, just find something that gets you moving and then get moving.

Fitness is addictive—in a good way. All of those feel-good chemicals like dopamine and serotonin released in your brain keep you coming back for more. You just have to start.

Simple things—things you can do every day—will increase your overall activity. They are no substitute for actually getting your heart rate going, but they will still make a difference. Park at the far end of the parking lot at the store and walk in. Turn the TV off and pick up a hobby. Learn to play an instrument. Start taking a martial arts or self-defense class.

Just get off the couch! If you do, you will soon find yourself wanting to do more and more as you begin to reap the benefits of movement.

As you continue to push your limits, you'll need to graduate to harder workouts. There is no shortage of options out there. Your local gym has weights and cardio rooms. There are group fitness classes springing up all over the place. There are tons of options. When Tracy and I met she was doing Paula Abdul and Cindy Crawford workout tapes. I was taking martial arts classes and working out at the Y. The kids and I all do martial arts together. They are also all involved in gymnastics. Our oldest plays baseball.

For the past 12 years, we have been been doing at-home workout programs almost exclusively. It's just easier and more convenient for us. You've got plenty of options for at-home workouts, even more so with the growing trend of streaming services. You don't even need a DVD player. All you need is a smartphone, a tablet or a streaming service like AppleTV or Roku or Amazon Fire. It's often less expensive and less time consuming to workout at home. We are a busy people. In the time it takes most people to drive to and from the gym, you can be done with your workout and getting on with your day.

Whatever you decide, do your research. If you opt to go to the gym, find a certified trainer to help you develop a program. If you opt to workout at home, find a streaming service or DVD program with good reviews and proven success stories.

As you are looking for programs, keep in mind that fitness is multi-faceted. There are several components to fitness, and all of them are important. In his book, *Bring It!*, Tony Horton says that variety is the spice of fitness. It is the first of his 11 Laws of Health and Fitness.[49] That means you need to mix up your workouts because when you do "the same type of exercise over and over, with no variation in activity, you increase your risk of overuse injuries and ailments such as tendinitis."[50]

There are five basic components of fitness: muscular strength, muscular endurance, cardiovascular endurance, flexibility, and body fat composition. In addition to these five, there are three performance components that I believe are also important: balance, agility, and coordination.

You may have noticed that most of these components of fitness have nothing to do with appearance. Fitness is not about how you look; it's about how well you are able to perform even basic everyday tasks. We discipline our bodies so they can serve us and serve God.

Bottom line—train hard so you can be fully alive.

CHAPTER 10

THE PILLAR OF FOCUS

Do not conform to the pattern of this world, but be transformed by the renewing of your mind.
—THE APOSTLE PAUL (Romans 12:2 NIV)

The successful warrior is the average man, with laser-like focus.[1]
—BRUCE LEE

I don't care how much power, brilliance or energy you have, if you don't harness it and focus it on a specific target, and hold it there you're never going to accomplish as much as your ability warrants.[2]
— ZIG ZIGLAR

We become what we focus on. I know, that sounds silly, and there was a time when I would have written off a statement like that as new-age mumbo jumbo. But that is exactly what God tells us in His Word. Think about it, how many times does the Bible tell us to meditate (focus) on the things of God? I count at least 13 (Joshua 1:8; Psalms 1:2; 63:6; 77:6, 12; 119:15, 23, 27, 48, 78, 148; 143:5; 145:5). Philippians 4:8 says to "Fix your thoughts on what is true, and honorable, and right, and pure, and lovely, and admirable. Think about things that are excellent and worthy of praise" (NLT). The New American Standard translation tells us to "dwell on these things," and the New King James says to "meditate" on them. That makes 14.

In an incredibly beautiful passage. Paul told the Corinthians, "And we all, who with unveiled faces contemplate the Lord's glory, are being transformed into his image with ever-increasing glory, which comes from the Lord, who is the Spirit." (2 Corinthians 3:18 NIV). That's a little poetic, but what he was saying is that as we focus our gaze upon the glory of God through the ministry of the Spirit, we are gradually transformed into the same image. We are regaining some of what was distorted in the fall—the fullness of the image of God in us.

Call it what you want, but there is a principle—a law—that says we tend to become like what we mediate and focus on. In the Western world, we tend to think of this in terms of mental focus. That's why Paul, in writing to the church at Rome says, "be transformed by the renewing of your mind" (Romans 12:1-2). But this level of thinking goes deeper. Meditation happens in the heart.

If your desire is to not just improve your health temporarily, but to create lasting change, you will need to focus both your mind and your heart.

FOCUSING YOUR MIND

Every January 1, millions of Americans make a "resolution" to eat better, to start working out regularly, and to improve their health. I've done it. I'm fairly confident you have too. And within a few weeks, 75 percent of us have given up. In the end only 8 percent will succeed.[3] It's a rather sad indictment, but it's true. You and I both know that by February 1 the gyms are empty again, the food at the typical football watch party would give an elephant a heart attack, and the overwhelming majority of people continue on their slow downward spiral.

On the bright side, there is that 8 percent of people who do manage to turn their lives around. Have you ever wondered about the difference between those who succeed and those who fail? When I was a member of the majority who quit, I thought that those dedicated few had some sort of genetic advantage. Well, they had an advantage all right, but it had nothing to do with genetics.

It had everything to do with vision.

What is a resolution anyway? According to the dictionary, it is "a firm decision to do or not to do something."[4] A firm decision? Not with a 92 percent failure rate. More like wishful thinking. When you make a decision, you literally leave yourself no other option.

Here's a fun fact to illustrate what I mean: When you see words that end in some form of "-cide" and "-cise," they usually have something to do with killing or cutting. For example, "incise" means to "cut into something," while "precision" means to "cut off before (shorten)." So, decide and decision mean to "cut off" or "kill off." A *firm* decision, then, should mean completely severing every other option—no going back. Think of it as a sacred vow.

When we decide it is time to take our health seriously, we usually start by setting goals. For example, you may set a goal to lose a certain amount of weight or to get into a certain size. Maybe you want to run your first 5k or to do a certain number of push-ups or pull-ups. Maybe you're like my dad, whose first goal was simply to walk 50 yards without having to stop because he was in so much pain.

No matter how big or small, we all start with a goal in mind. Once we have those goals in place, we then adjust our behavior to achieve them—at least that's how it works in theory. But for 90 percent of us, something happens along the way that gets us off track. So, the real question is, *How do we stay on course?*

WHERE DO YOU WANT TO BE?

There is a fun little dialogue in Lewis Carroll's *Alice in Wonderland* when Alice comes to a fork in the road and is trying to decide which way to go. It is at this point that she meets the Cheshire Cat, so she asks him for advice—she asks him which way she should go from there. The Cat tells her it depends on where she wants to get to. When Alice responds that she doesn't care, the Cat wisely responds that in that case it really doesn't matter which way she goes. Alice tries to explain herself by saying that she just wants to get *somewhere*, to which the Cat responds, "Oh, you're sure to do that if only you walk long enough."

In his unique way, the Cheshire Cat was telling Alice that before you can know which path to take, you need to know where you want to go.

Proverbs 29:18 tells us, "Where there is no vision, the people perish" (KJV). Although the King James Version is probably the version we hear quoted most, I love the way newer translations put it: "Where there is no prophetic vision the people cast off restraint" (ESV).

Notice how it underscores "where there is no *prophetic* vision" (emphasis added). In other words, we don't see God's vision for what He wants to do in your life. We don't see His hope and His direction, so we "cast off restraint." Without God's vision, we become undisciplined and unfocused. We do whatever feels good at the moment. But the result is a slow death—we perish.

We have to know where we are going and how to get there because life is a continuous series of crossroads. According to multiple internet sources, an adult makes about 35,000 remotely conscious decisions a day. That sounds outlandish, right? But there it is. And then you have to consider that researchers at Cornell University found that we make 226.7

decisions every day related to food alone.[5] And each one of these decisions leads us off in a different direction.

Each choice comes at the sacrifice of the other choice. Some decisions make a relatively small difference, while some make a big difference. But all of them change the trajectory of our life in one way or another. Even the smallest decisions matter because they compound. They work together over the course of a day, a week, a year, a decade, which means the long-term effect is exponential.

If you don't have a clear picture of where you are going, how can you make the right choice in the moment? Our God-given vision provides a plan so that we can make the right choices as we face various situations.

Now, let's get personal for a moment. What exactly is your vision for your life? When I first read Steven Furtick's book *Sun Stand Still* in 2011, it challenged me, convicted me, encouraged me, and emboldened me to live with God-sized purpose. I didn't even make it through the first chapter without God grabbing my heart and driving me to my knees. As much as God has done in my life and through me in the lives of others, I was still thinking too small. It brought me to tears and lit a fire under me to live an audacious life.

Early in the book, Furtick wrote:

If you ever encounter a theology that doesn't directly connect the greatness of God with your potential to do great things on his behalf, it's not biblical theology. File it under heresy. I'll take that further: if you're not daring to believe God for the impossible, you're sleeping through some of the best parts of your Christian life. And further still: if the size of your vision for your life isn't intimidating to you, there's a good chance it's insulting to God."[6]

He's absolutely right—every fiber of my being told me so. Right then and there, I had to ask God to forgive how my lack of vision and faith was insulting to Him. God did not put us on His earth to live ordinary, safe lives. The same power that allowed Jesus and the apostles to perform miracles and raised Christ from the dead resides in us. For my part, I am not satisfied to live an ordinary life! I know and believe that God can and will do great things through me. And I'm trusting him to touch thousands of lives, even millions, through me. Not because I am so great, but because He is! "But we have this treasure in jars of clay, to show that the surpassing power belongs to God and not to us" (2 Corinthians 4:7 ESV).

What about you? How big is your vision for what God can do through your life? Are you tired of living an "ordinary" life? Do you find yourself frustrated, knowing that there is more to life than survival, knowing that you were created to live fully and abundantly? This book is an invitation to step out in faith and join me on this journey. If you have never asked God what He wants to do through you, I highly recommend you do that before you do anything else.

I am confident "that he who began a good work in [us] will bring it to completion at the day of Jesus Christ" (Philippians 1:6 ESV). Trust your Father to lead you into this great adventure called life, knowing He is in control. Take His hand and take that first step.

ALIGNING YOUR GOALS WITH YOUR LIFE

Throughout my life I have had mentors stress the importance of setting goals and of having a focused mindset. I have read books, listened to trainings, and attended seminars from some of the greatest success coaches out there: John Maxwell, Dave Ramsey, Zig Ziglar, Brian Tracy, Chalene Johnson, and a host of others. One day during a call with one of my mentors, PJ McClure, we were talking about a recent group I had participated in where we were all focused on a particular business goal. This group included trainings by some of the top earners in our company. It was great material.

But while everyone in the group had the same goal and the same training, only about 4 percent of us hit our goal. I was about to start a similar group for my team, but wanted to figure out how to help a higher percentage of them achieve their goals. As we were talking, PJ asked me what the disconnect was in the original group. What kept everyone from hitting their goal? The training wasn't the problem. The goal itself wasn't the problem. So what was?

We hired PJ to do a series of short videos as a way to set up the members of our group for greater success. In the first video, PJ used a millstone to explain what was going on.

A millstone, he said, is only as useful as the context it is used in. For thousands of years, millstones were a central part of society; but in our modern age, we have lost touch with what a millstone is. It's a big rock. Technically, it is a large round stone, weighing almost a ton, that was used to grind grain. In that context, it is life-giving and good. But there is a flip side. Most of us know what a millstone is from Jesus' quote in Matthew 18:6, it's better to "have a large millstone hung around their neck and to be drowned in the depths of the sea" than to cause a little child of God to fall into sin. That's a bad deal.

That phrase is the basis of the secondary definition of millstone—"a heavy burden." In proper context, a millstone is good and useful and life-enhancing. Out of context, it is a heavy burden or even life-stealing. Goals work the same way. A goal is only as useful as the context it's set in. A goal out of context is a goal set without any consideration of how it fits into the rest of your life. When you set a goal out of context, it becomes a burden. You either won't achieve it, or achieve it and not be able to hold on to it, or achieve it and suffer in other areas of your life.

This should go without saying, but your goals need to be *your* goals. Goals can neither be borrowed nor given. They have to be personal. People often ask if I can help one of their friends or family members. Usually, it's a wife asking if I can help her husband. (Note to the men, our wives do this because they love us and want us around longer, not because they are trying to "fix" us). My answer is always the same: I will be glad to talk with them; but unless it's something they want and are committed to achieving, it's out of my hands. If you start trying to pursue something as important as improving your health and fitness, and you're doing it because of what someone else wants and not because it's what you want, you are going to end up frustrated at best.

When I'm talking with a potential client about their goals, they often say things like, "I want to lose ____ pounds" or "I want to look like this person" or "I want to be this size" or "I want more energy" or, in my friend Sarah's case, "I want to be fully alive." Regardless of what they tell me about their goal, I always begin with the same response: *Great! Tell me why.*

KNOWING YOUR WHY

Asking why allows you to discover where—or even if—your goal fits into the context of your vision for your life. It's a very simple question, but most people never ask it—and that's why they fail. Living an optimal God-honoring, healthy lifestyle is not easy. Nothing about the Christian walk is. Habits cannot be broken; they must be replaced by new ones. That requires working through an uncomfortable period. As Dr. Denis Waitley said, "Habits are like submarines. They run silent and deep. They also are like comfortable beds, in that they're easy to get into, but difficult to get out of."[7]

You've probably heard it said that it takes 21 days to form a habit; and while that may be true, it sometimes takes months or even years to make the new habit permanent. Think about it, you've been you for a long time. You're not just adding something new—you're breaking down strongholds in your life. This is going to be hard. The sooner you wrap your mind around that, the better. Willpower alone won't last long enough for you to power through.

I love how Darren Hardy puts it, "Assuming willpower is what you need to change your habits is akin to trying to keep a hungry grizzly bear out of your picnic basket by covering it with a napkin. To fight the bear of your bad habits, you need something stronger."[8]

Maybe you thought you kept struggling to lose weight or eat better or start exercising because you lacked willpower. Not true. I had a woman once tell me that it was because she was lazy.

She was a very successful businesswoman and the mom of very responsible and well-behaved children, so I knew better. I asked her if she was lazy when it came to her business or her children.

"Oh, no," she said, "not at all."

"So it's not that you're lazy," I said with a smile. "You work very hard at what's important to you. You just haven't made your health important yet."

She had bought into a lie. Most of us have at one point or another. Like I had done for so many years, she believed her failure to lose weight and keep it off was the result of laziness and a lack of willpower. But it was neither. It was a matter of priorities.

Willpower will only get you so far. Willpower is limited and exhaustible. We have more willpower first thing in the morning than we do late at night because we use most of it up during the course of the day. Those 35,000 daily decisions take their toll. If you want to make significant changes in your life, like the ones required for being fully alive, you'll need something stronger. You'll need a bigger reason—something much deeper than "I want to look better" or "I want to lose weight."

Our actions are determined by deeply-held core values and beliefs. We may be able to make temporary changes, but we will always revert back to our old habits unless we can connect our new habits to those core beliefs and to the vision we have for our lives. It's not enough to want to be healthy and fit. You've got to know why it matters to you. Otherwise, you'll just revert back to your old habits.

You've got to have what Darren Hardy calls "why-power."[9] The power of your why is what gets you through the daily grind, the temptations of that slice of pizza or cake, the mornings where you don't feel like getting out of bed and working out, the days when you feel overwhelmed and just want to sit in front of the TV and eat a pint of ice cream. To bring it a little closer to home, allow me to share an analogy from Hardy that I use all of the time:

If I were to put a ten-inch-wide, thirty-foot-long plank on the ground and say, "If you walk the length of the plank, I'll give you twenty dollars," would you do it? Of course, it's an easy twenty bucks. But what if I took that same plank and made a roof-top "bridge" between two 100-story buildings? That same twenty dollars for walking the thirty-foot plank no longer looks desirable or even possible, does it? You'd look at me and say, "Not on your life." However, if your child was on the opposite building, and that building was on fire, would you walk the length of the plank to save him? Without question and immediately—you'd do it, twenty dollars or not. Why is it that the first time I asked you to cross that sky-high plank, you said no way, yet, the second time you wouldn't hesitate? The risks and the dangers are the same. What changed? Your why changed—your reason for wanting to do it. You see, when the reason is big enough, you will be willing to perform almost any how.[10]

I don't know how many times I've shared that analogy, but I still get choked up when I get to the part about your child being on the other building. I'm tearing up now just writing it. I think about my own kids. They are a big part of my why. There is something else hidden here. You'll never find your why in your head because it lives in your heart.

ENGAGING YOUR HEART

Somehow we have forgotten the central role our hearts play in our lives. We rely on reason and logic. We bury our feelings—at least we think we do. In reality, it is our hearts and not our minds that drive our decisions. It is impossible to consistently act in a way that is inconsistent with how we feel. The trick, then, is to get what we know in our minds to travel down and penetrate our hearts. But how do we do this?

It has been said that the greatest distance in the world is from the head to the heart. Nowhere is this truer than our faith. It's very easy to get caught up in having the right doctrines without ever really having our faith move into our heart. That's where we get into trouble. It is no accident that the Bible has so much to say about the heart, mentioning it nearly 300 times. The heart takes preeminence over knowledge, over faith, over obedience, over gifts, and over worship precisely because all of those things flow from the heart (Proverbs 4:23). Isn't that what Paul's famous treatise on love tells us, "the greatest of these is love" (1 Corinthians 13:1-13)? Love is the heart in action.

Head knowledge alone won't cut it. James wrote, "You believe that God is one; you do well. Even the demons believe—and shudder! Do you want to be shown, you foolish person, that faith apart from works is useless?" (James 2:19–20 ESV). Knowing is not enough to produce a changed life. It must capture our hearts.

Words alone also mean nothing. Jesus rebuked the scribes and Pharisees as hypocrites and quoted Isaiah, "This people honors me with their lips, but their heart is far from me" (Matthew 15:8 ESV). God doesn't care what we say. He cares about our heart.

Jesus said the greatest and foremost commandment is, "You shall love the Lord your God with all your heart and with all your soul and with all your mind" (Matthew 22:37 ESV). Notice he lists the heart first. Paul said, "For with the heart one believes and is justified" (Romans 10:10 ESV). It is not with the mind one believes, but with the heart.

And when it comes to persevering through difficulties, our logic and reason won't get us through, but our hearts. Paul encouraged us, "Therefore, having this ministry by the mercy of God, we do not lose heart. . . . We are afflicted in every way, but not crushed; perplexed, but not driven to despair; persecuted, but not forsaken; struck down, but not destroyed. . . . So we do not lose heart" (2 Corinthians 4:1, 8-9, 16 ESV).

When we give up on something, anything, whether it be a healthy eating resolution or exercise plan or a job or a relationship, what do we say? *My heart wasn't in it.* If we want to succeed at anything in life, we must find a way to engage both our hearts and minds. In an article about connecting our hearts and minds, John Piper said:

> Jesus meant for truth in the head to waken passion in the heart: "You will know the truth, and the truth will set you free" (John 8:32). Free from sin. Free from what Paul calls "deceitful desires" (Ephesians 4:22) into a new world of holy passions. The apostle Paul demanded the same thing: "felt truth." "They did not welcome the love of the truth so as to be saved" (2 Thessalonians 2:10). Not just: They did not welcome the truth; but more: They did not welcome the love of the truth. The truth was not felt as beautiful and precious.[11]

How profound! Jesus intended that the truth we store in the head make a difference in our hearts. What we know should influence what we do— and how we do it. That's focus!

The human mind is a lot like a computer. It is great at receiving and processing information. It is a wonderfully magnificent machine; but like any machine, it can be detached and indifferent. As Eldredge said:

[The mind] is a beautiful gift of God. Why, you are using your mind even now on your search for God and for life. But it remains, for the most part, indifferent. Your mind tells you that it is now 2:00 A.M. and your daughter has not returned, for the car is not in the driveway. Your heart wrestles with whether or not it is cause for worry.[12]

The heart and mind are meant to work together. The mind handles surface level information and calculations, but the heart does our deepest thinking. We meditate on things in our heart. The thoughts of our heart determine who we are. Yes, I said the *thoughts* of our heart. Actually, God said it, not me: "As [a man] thinks in his heart, so is he" (NKJV).

The mind holds knowledge, but the heart stores wisdom. Two-thirds of the Book of Proverbs was written and collected by Solomon. You may recall that when Solomon became king, God told him to ask for one thing—anything—and the request would be granted. What did Solomon ask for? An "understanding heart" (1 Kings 3:9 NASB). This pleased God so much that He not only gave Solomon "a wise and discerning heart, so that there has been no one like you before you, nor shall one like you arise after you" (1 Kings 3:12 NASB), but He also gave him riches and honor.

Our hearts give us the courage to do things that are difficult and intimidating, and courage gives us the will to endure any hardship. In fact, courage comes from the heart, literally. The word itself comes from the Old French *corage*, which is rooted in the Latin *cor,* meaning "heart."[13] Even if you didn't know that, you probably understood it. Jesus said, "I have said these things to you, that in me you may have peace. In the world you will have tribulation. But take heart; I have overcome the world" (John 16:33 ESV). Take heart. Have courage.

Your heart provides the courage to cross that plank suspended 100 stories off the ground to rescue your child from the burning building. That's not a rational decision. Your mind tells you all of the reasons not to go, but your heart tells you you have to. In the words of Hannibal, "I will find a way or I will make one!"[14]

It is where we meditate on things. It is where we ponder.

And you thought the heart was purely emotional.

The day my doctor told me I had high blood pressure and high cholesterol and pre-diabetes, my mind processed the information. I knew I needed to eat better and exercise. Knowing wasn't the problem. It wasn't until that knowledge intersected with my dad's question, "Who's going to raise your boys when you're gone?" that my heart got involved. I was emotionally invested from that point on.

My mind and heart were both focused on change. I found my "why-power;" and for the first time in my life, I followed through on changing my habits. It didn't take long for me to blow right past what I thought my goal was. I achieved a level of health and vitality I didn't even know existed.

BEWARE THE THIEF

Remember in John 10:10 where Jesus tells us that He came to give life to the fullest? And just before that, He warned us about a thief who would try to steal that life. That enemy takes great pleasure not in taking it by force, but by convincing us to give it up. He does that through deceit and manipulation. He lies and leads us to doubt God. That was how he attacked our first parents. He lied to Eve—and Adam. He questioned God's Word by suggesting that God was holding back on them. He convinced them they wouldn't really face the consequences of eating the forbidden fruit. Eve and Adam fell for it, and here we are in a fallen and broken world.

It worked the first time so he's had no reason to change tactics. Jesus said, "He was a murderer from the beginning, and does not stand in the truth, because there is no truth in him. When he lies, he speaks out of his own character, for he is a liar and the father of lies" (John 8:44 ESV).

Unless we are awake and aware, it's easy to buy into his lies. It would be much easier if he came to us in the caricature of the guy in the red suit with the horns and pitchfork, but he doesn't. He's much more subtle than that. He "disguises himself as an angel of light" (2 Corinthians 11:14 ESV). He whispers in our ear, and we think the voice is our own.

John Eldridge tells the story of a friend of his who decided to get into shape.

> My friend Aaron decided to get into shape. He went out and took a run. First, the Enemy tried discouragement to get him to quit. *Look how far you have to go. You can't do this— you'll die out there. Give it up.* Aaron thought, *Gee—it is a long way. I'm not sure I can do this.* But then he recognized what was going on and pressed into it. The attack became more personal, more vicious. He was running along, and he was hearing stuff like this: *You're just a fat pig. You always have been.* A gorgeous woman in fabulous shape approached from the other direction. *She'd never be attracted to a slob like you.* "By the time I got back to my car," he said, "it felt like I'd been assaulted. But this time, I knew what it was and I won. I made no agreements."[15]

Sounds kind of like my friend who bought into the lie and agreed with the enemy that she was lazy. Once you recognize the lie, you still have to fight it. This is a battle for your heart and mind; and your enemy is not so easily thwarted. But take heart, Jesus has already overcome him (John 16:33; 1 John 4:4).

The enemy is tricky. Often, he'll even co-opt other people into assisting him. That was true for my mom. Growing up, she heard her mother consistently tell her she was fat. So she began to see herself as fat—that became her identity and it's something she still struggles with. I don't think her mom was trying to be malicious, but that doesn't matter. The devil was behind the lie and *his* intent is malicious. Always.

I promise you, you'll come across people in your life who will not be happy about your decision to improve your health. Some will tell you that you are missing out on enjoying food. It's a lie. You'll enjoy food more.

Some will tell you that you're looking underweight. It's a lie. Everyone else is overweight.

Some will tell you that time spent working out robs you of time you could spend doing something else. It's a lie. Working out gives you more time. I love the cartoon where the doctor asks his patient, "So what fits your busy schedule better, working out an hour a day or being dead twenty-four?"

They will tell you you're being selfish and vain. It's a lie. You're being disciplined and honoring God in your body. They're being selfish because misery loves company.

I know you'll hear these lies because I have heard them—usually from well-meaning people who simply didn't know better. Kind of like Peter when he rebuked Jesus for saying He would have to suffer and die and rise again on the third day. Jesus recognized who was behind the rebuke: "Get behind me, Satan! You are a hindrance to me" (Matthew 16:23 ESV).

Now, I don't recommend you say that to your friends and family, but it's good to recognize the source of their antagonism.

I wish I could tell you it gets easier. It doesn't, but you do get stronger the more you flex the muscles of your heart and mind. Stay focused on your health goals and why they matter to you. Write them down. Follow through on your plans. Eat Clean. Train Hard. Live Passionately. Journal about your journey.

Oh, don't attempt this journey on your own. You're going to need a fellowship.

CHAPTER 11

THE PILLAR OF FELLOWSHIP

Fate has chosen him.
A Fellowship will protect him.
Evil will hunt them.[1]
> — THE FELLOWSHIP OF THE RING (Theatrical
> Trailer)

You might remember that the first Christians were called "followers of the Way" (Acts 9: 2; 18: 25– 26). They had found the Way of Life and had given themselves over to it. They lived together, ate together, fought together, celebrated together. They were intimate allies; it was a fellowship of the heart. How wonderful it would be if we could find the same. How dangerous it will be if we do not.[2]
> — JOHN ELDREDGE

As iron sharpens iron, so a friend sharpens a friend.
> — PROVERBS 27:17 NLT

Therefore encourage one another and build one another up.
> — 1 THESSALONIANS 5:11 ESV

You may remember a classic scene from Peter Jackson's adaptation of Tolkein's, *The Fellowship of the Ring:*

The peace and serenity of their surroundings is interrupted by an argument between members of the council. As the argument grows louder and more heated, one of the little ones, a hobbit, sees a vision that terrifies him. He knows what has to be done and a look of determination sets on his face. Suddenly, Frodo stands and speaks in a strong, clear voice., "I will take it! . . . I will take it!"

Gandalf, the old and wise wizard, hearing the courage in the voice of the hobbit, closes his eyes. The argument dies down as the members of the council all turn to see who is speaking. "I will take the Ring to Mordor," says Frodo. Stunned silence. Frodo looks around the courtyard at the astonished faces and continues, "Though . . . I do not know the way."

Gandalf approaches Frodo and places his hands reassuringly on Frodo's shoulders, "I will help you bear this burden, Frodo Baggins, as long as it is yours to bear."

Aragorn stands and proclaims, "If by my life or death, I can protect you, I will." He walks over to Frodo and kneels before him adding, "You have my sword."

Legolas joins in, "And you have my bow," followed by Gimli who shouts, "And my axe!"

Boromir looks at them all then walks towards Frodo. "You carry the fate of us all little one," he says, "If this is indeed the will of the Council, then Gondor will see it done."

Frodo stares in wonder as the Greatest Warriors in all Middle Earth stand at his side.

Sam, who has been unseen up to this point jumps up from behind the bushes and shouts, "Here! Mister Frodo is not goin' anywhere without me!"

An amused look spreads across Lord Elrond's face. "No, indeed," he says, "It is hardly possible to separate you . . . even when he is summoned to a secret council and you are not."

At this point, Pippin and Merry run out from their hiding place behind the pillars and shout, "Wait! We are coming too!" Merry says, "You'd have to send us home tied up in a sack to stop us!" Pippin adds, "Anyway . . . you need people of intelligence on this sort of mission . . . quest . . . thing." To which Merry quips, "Well that rules you out, Pip."

Lord Elrond surveys the group assembled before him and proclaims, "Nine companions . . . So be it! You shall be the Fellowship of the Ring!"³

Have I mentioned how indebted I am to John Eldredge for his words and his ministry? I have yet to meet him; but when I do, I will embrace him as a mentor and brother-in-arms. We share a love of epic books and movies. Our hearts burn with a desire to live for God with passion and purpose and encourage others in the journey.

Of all of the amazing books John has written, the two that have the greatest impact on my life and how I live it are *Wild at Heart* and *Waking the Dead*. When it comes to this idea of the importance—the absolute necessity of having a fellowship of the heart to make it through life—you'll never find a more ardent and compelling synopsis than the introduction to chapter 11 of *Waking the Dead*.

Once more, lend a mythic eye to your situation. Let your heart ponder this:

You awake to find yourself in the midst of a great and terrible war. It is, in fact, our most desperate hour. Your King and dearest Friend calls you forth. Awake, come fully alive, your good heart set free and blazing for him and for those yet to be rescued. You have a glory that is needed. You are given a quest, a mission that will take you deep into the heart of the kingdom of darkness, to break down gates of bronze and cut through bars of iron so that your people might be set free from their bleak prisons. He asks that you heal them. Of course, you will face many dangers; you will be hunted.

Would you try to do this alone?

Something stronger than fate has chosen you. Evil will hunt you. And so a fellowship must protect you. Honestly, though he is a very brave and true hobbit, Frodo hasn't a chance without Sam, Merry, Pippin, Gandalf, Aragorn, Legolas, and Gimli. He has no real idea what dangers and trials lie ahead. The dark mines of Moria; the Balrog that awaits him there; the evil orcs called the Urak-hai that will hunt him; the wastes of the Emyn Muil. He will need his friends. And you will need yours. You must cling to those you have; you must search wide and far for those you do not yet have. You must not go alone. From the beginning, right there in Eden, the Enemy's strategy has relied upon a simple aim: divide and conquer. Get them isolated, and take them out.

When Neo is set free from the Matrix, he joins the crew of the Nebuchadnezzar— the little hovercraft that is the headquarters and ship of the small fellowship called to set the captives free. There are nine of them in all, each a character in his own way, but nonetheless a company of the heart, a "band of brothers," a family bound together in a single fate. Together, they train for battle. Together, they plan their path. When they go back into the Matrix to set others free, each one has a role, a gifting, a glory. They function as a team. And they watch each other's back. Neo is fast, really fast, but he still would have been taken out if it hadn't been for Trinity. Morpheus is more gifted than them all, but it took the others to rescue him.

You see this sort of thing at the center of every great story. Dorothy takes her journey with the Scarecrow, the Tin Woodman, the Lion, and of course, Toto. Prince Caspian is joined by the last few faithful Narnians, and together they overthrow the wicked king Miraz. Though in the eyes of the world they are only gladiator-slaves, walking dead men, Maximus rallies his little band and triumphs over the greatest empire on earth. When Captain John Miller is sent deep behind enemy lines to save Private Ryan, he goes in with a squad of eight rangers. And, of course, Jesus had the Twelve. This is written so deeply on our hearts: You must not go alone. The Scriptures are full of such warnings, but until we see our desperate situation, we hear it as an optional religious assembly for an hour on Sunday mornings.

Think again of Frodo or Neo or Caspian or Jesus. Imagine you are surrounded by a small company of friends who know you well (characters, to be sure, but they love you, and you have come to love them). They understand that we all are at war, know that the purposes of God are to bring a man or a woman fully alive, and are living by sheer necessity and joy in the Four Streams. They fight for you, and you for them. Imagine you could have a little fellowship of the heart. Would you want it if it were available?[4]

God intended for us to live in community, just as He does within the Trinity. Jesus prays for us to be one just as He is one with the Father (John 17:21). We see a wonderful picture of this in the New Testament Church. Luke, the physician and author of both Luke and Acts, tells us "All the believers were united in heart and mind" (Acts 4:32 NLT). There was a very special bond going on there. It went beyond just getting together for a meal or to socialize. It's what the New Testament writers meant when they talked about church.

I love our church! We are part of the Journey Fellowship campus of Oak Hills Church in San Antonio. I love our teaching pastors, Max Lucado and Randy Frazee. I love the worship. I love being part of the worship team. I love volunteering with the student ministry. I love the friends we see every week. Being involved in the Sunday service every week is an integral part of our lives and our walk with Christ. It is not, however, where community happens.

Community happens in our small group.

Oak Hills knows this, which is why they encourage and equip us to go into our community to lead and participate in neighborhood small groups. Our small group is amazing! We sit close together in the worship services, hang out together, share meals, and pray together. We dig deeper into God's Word together, and we share our struggles and celebrate victories together. We also all happen to be committed to healthy living, so we share recipes. We get out and go to parks and on hikes together. Our children play together. We do life together.

The New Testament Greek word for this is *koinonia*. It is translated "fellowship."

The truth is we *need* fellowship. That's right . . . it's not a *want*; it's a *need*. As God said, it's not good for us to be alone. He tells us:

"Two people are better off than one, for they can help each other succeed. If one person falls, the other can reach out and help. But someone who falls alone is in real trouble. Likewise, two people lying close together can keep each other warm. But how can one be warm alone? A person standing alone can be attacked and defeated, but two can stand back-to-back and conquer. Three are even better, for a triple-braided cord is not easily broken." (Ecclesiastes 4:9–12 NLT)

INTENTIONAL FELLOWSHIP

Fellowships require work. They don't just happen, so you're going to have to be intentional about it. You're going to have to fight to find one and then fight to keep it together. Even the Fellowship of the Ring was divided for a time. It actually worked out because they had different roles to play in the unfolding epic. But no member was ever alone, and they were always together in heart, even when hurtful things were said and done.

Sometimes it's easy to buy into the thinking that it would be easier to go it alone—except it's not. That's another lie the enemy whispers so he can isolate you and take you out. There is no such thing as "Lone Ranger Christianity." After all, even the Lone Ranger wasn't alone—he had Tonto. Just like Frodo had Sam.

The best example, of course, is Jesus. Our Lord surrounded Himself with a fellowship and developed deep relationships. He called the 12 disciples; and within that, He had an inner circle of Peter, James and John. He took these three with Him into the garden of Gethsemane to pray in His hour of greatest need. He knew what was coming. He knew he would have to finish His mission alone. But He still wanted His band of brothers with Him.

They didn't understand the gravity of the moment and fell asleep on the job. They were unable to see the battle raging all around them. They could not grasp the depth of the darkness that was coming. Jesus knew and asked them to stay with Him, to keep watch and pray. He knew He was headed into battle.

And that is precisely why we need one another. We're at war too.

The phrase "one another" occurs 100 times in the New Testament, and 59 of those are exhortations to the Church concerning interpersonal relationships.[5] Call it a blueprint for fellowship. "One another" is two words in English; but in the Greek of the New Testament, it is just one word — *allelon*. *Allelon* is the genitive plural of *allos,* "another." We don't usually concern ourselves with grammatical details, but this is an interesting case. The genitive case is the Greek equivalent of our possessive case because it often identifies one noun as possessing another noun.[6]

The idea is that we belong to one another. Paul confirmed this idea by reminding us, "so we, though many, are one body in Christ, and individually members one of another" (Romans 12:5 ESV, see also Ephesians 4:25). This is a pretty big deal. So big that it prompted Andy Stanley to say, "The primary activity of the church was one-anothering one another."[7]

We are told to love one another (20 times), to bear with one another, to carry one another's burdens, to encourage one another, to serve one another, to instruct one another, to forgive one another. We are told to "think of ways to motivate one another to acts of love and good works" (Hebrews 10:24 NLT). And here's the real kicker—Jesus said serving each other is the key to greatness.

One day the disciples were arguing among themselves about which one of them would be the greatest in Christ's kingdom. How dare they, right? Actually, Jesus doesn't rebuke them for this. Instead, he tells them how to accomplish it. He sat them down and told them, "Whoever wants to be first must take last place and be the servant of everyone else" (Mark 9:35 NLT).

If you're thinking that's all easier said than done, you're right, but it's also essential to life—a full life. That's why the Bible talks so much about it. That's why we have to be intentional about it.

THE OBESITY EPIDEMIC AND THE CHURCH

Our nation is facing a health crisis. The obesity epidemic claims a million or more lives every year through heart disease, strokes, cancer, diabetes, and other complications. Millions more are being robbed of quality of life. God wants to bring healing to a sick and dying world, and He always works through His people to accomplish His will. We have been called. Will you answer the call?

When I first began teaching these principles as a ministry, it was at TLC Church in Memphis. Dana had asked me to teach our Wednesday night Bible studies. I was fortunate that I had his backing and blessing, but I also knew that plenty of people were more than a little skeptical. Before Bible study we always shared a meal together. The main course was catered by a local Italian restaurant—with dishes like spaghetti or lasagna. Church members would bring potluck sides and desserts.

The first night I taught, it was lasagna. The following Wednesday when I walked in, it was grilled chicken and sautéed spinach.

That wasn't my call. God convicted hearts, and the change was made without my knowledge. But it was a proud moment. God was using me to make a difference. Now, in all fairness, not everything that members brought was healthy, but we were making progress. Church members, like Mike, began asking me for help. It was a start.

Not long after that first series, Dan Henley, pastor of a sister church called Journey Christian Church, asked me to speak to his congregation. That was fun. The congregation of TLC was primarily Caucasian, while the congregation of Journey was primarily African-American. Dana and Dan both had a vision to foster racial reconciliation in Memphis. It was incredible.

Journey was a lively church; and if you aren't familiar with the culture of black churches, the congregation will often talk to you while you're speaking. You can imagine it got talkative when we started talking about food. I loved it! We had a great time of studying Scriptures together. It was a blessing.

TLC and Journey partnered together to host a weekly Fit Club at the Journey Campus. We would get together once a week and put a workout DVD in and move together. We would have "biggest loser" type contests with weekly weigh-ins and celebrate progress together. People were encouraging and cheering each other on. We even made the local news.

A reporter for WMCTV named Daniel Hight had been one of my students when I was leading college ministry and reached out for help when he wanted to get in shape. As a reporter, he wanted to look good on camera and had decided he wanted to do a story about his own experience going through the Insanity program. When his final report aired, Daniel came out to Journey and did a story on our Fit Club on a night we were doing an Insanity® workout. We were able to share what our churches were doing to help reverse the trend of obesity in what had just been named the most obese city in the country. It was a great outreach into the community and a great way to bring people together.

Whatever small group we are a part of, we try to influence for the better. The small group we lead in our house now has transformed over time. When we get together, we always "break bread" together because that's a part of fellowshipping. Like us, another family brought healthy and delicious dishes because their children have GI issues and food allergies.

But we started a trend. Other families were inspired to bring healthier food. So, it's amazing and delicious and healthy all at once.

We are constantly looking for new recipes to share and try out. We invite people over to our house to workout with us. We go on hikes together with our families. A few of them have asked me about the Ultimate Reset that Tracy and I just went through recently. In fact, we'll be leading our group through a Reset and walking through this book together. Through this journey, they will be helping to develop a companion study guide that other small groups can use.

It's a model that has been proven over and over. My friend, Steve Willis, did it in his church. When Rick Warren did it at Saddleback, *The Daniel Plan* was born. Churches use this model for Dave Ramsey's *Financial Peace University*, for marriage classes, for discipleship classes. We grow in fellowships.

FINDING YOUR FELLOWSHIP

So how do you go about finding a fellowship that will journey with you on your quest to a healthy, God-honoring life? God promises that He will always provide a way for us. It is His will for you to glorify Him in your body and in your choices. You can start by asking Him to bring the right people to you. I promise, He will answer. Look around your church or small group for people who are interested in getting healthier. Talk to your neighbors and co-workers.

You can find virtual groups online. Actually, even if you have a local fellowship, setting up an online group for your fellowship is a great way to stay connected consistently. Tracy and I run online groups all the time with our local small groups, but we also connect with people all over the country and even some internationally. We set up groups on Facebook or through a Challenge Tracker app. We do group Zoom calls, and we post sweaty post-workout pics and recipes. We put up motivational posts, and we are always there to encourage each other and answer questions.

You've got to be intentional about this, but you will find people who will be there for you to support you in your goals. You may also need to distance yourself from those who are not supportive. Even if you only find one other person, that's enough. Like Frodo and Sam, you will still have each other, and you will have God. As Jesus promised, "For where two or three are gathered in my name, there am I among them" (Matthew 18:20 ESV).

The Foundation of Faith and the Pillar of Fellowship are the bookends of success. That's because they hold the others together. They are also the two that are most often missed. Most of us know on some level that we should eat better and that we should exercise more, even if we don't know why. And there is an increasing awareness of the power of setting goals and focusing the mind, although they still need to engage the heart.

But Faith gets missed because, well, most people have never made the connection between faith and fitness. Fellowship gets missed because we struggle with engaging in true fellowship. We might find a workout buddy to meet us at the gym or to go with us to Weight Watchers, but that's barely scratching the surface. Have I mentioned that this is war? A really cool thing happens to people who have experienced combat together. They develop a bond on a level that you just can't understand unless you've experienced it.

We need more of that in the church.

With your Fellowship at your side, you will find the strength to make the necessary lifestyle changes to put the Pillars of Food, Fitness and Focus in place. That's how you build a temple that will stand for a lifetime. And the best part is, with your fellowship, you will find joy in the journey. You will be able to do more together and serve more. You will be a mighty force to bring the Kingdom of God to earth. As Jesus taught us to pray to our Heavenly Father, "Your kingdom come, your will be done on earth as it is in heaven" (Matthew 6:10).

CONTAGIOUS HABITS

Did your parents or grandparents ever say things like, "You are who you hang out with?" Mine did. All the time. It turns out they were right. One of the biggest factors in determining how successful you will be in any area of your life is the people you spend the most time with—your fellowship. Success coach and speaker Jim Rohn has been credited with saying, "You are the average of the five people you spend the most time with." You will have the average of their relationships, their health, their income, and their attitudes. Look around you, is that true?

Whether or not it is true in other areas of life, it is certainly true when it comes to your health. It turns out that healthy (or unhealthy) behaviors are contagious. In 2007, *The New England Journal of Medicine* (*NEJM*) ran an article on an obesity study conducted by researchers at Harvard University and the University of California, San Diego. The study analyzed a large social network of 12,067 people over the course of 32 years (1971–2003). Here are a few fun statistics based on more than three decades of research:

- You are 37 percent more likely to be obese if your spouse is obese.
- You are 40 percent more likely to be obese if your sibling is obese.
- You are 57 percent more likely to be obese if your friends are obese.[8]

Turns out the company you keep is more powerful than genetics when it comes to obesity. Of course, a number of factors come into play here. For instance, when we surround ourselves with overweight people, it alters what we perceive as the norm. When I lost weight and people started telling me I was getting too thin, my thought was always, *No, everyone else you know is just overweight.*

We also are influenced by the food choices of our friends. If you go out to eat with a friend, and they order something healthy, you are more likely to do the same. True story: I was meeting a friend for lunch one day, and I found out later from his wife that when we set the lunch date he told her, "If I'm meeting Deryl for lunch, I'm going to have to eat something healthy." Her response—"Maybe you should eat with Deryl more often." I love it!

You tend to become like the people you hang out with the most. This wisdom has been around for millennia. "Become wise by walking with the wise; hang out with fools and watch your life fall to pieces" (Proverbs 13:20 MSG). And, "Do not be deceived: 'Bad company ruins good morals'" (1 Corinthians 15:33 ESV).

Not only do our friends influence us, but we also influence them. The NEJM study found that the greatest degree of influence existed between mutual, close friends. In those cases, when one person became obese, the other had a 171 percent greater chance of becoming obese as well. Furthermore, the study found that the ripple effect of a weight gain was significant out to three degrees of separation. That means if one person gains weight, their friends, and their friends' friends, and the next layer of friends past that also have a significantly greater chance of gaining weight. Habits are contagious.

The good news is that this also works in reverse. You are an influencer. As you start taking your health seriously and making better choices, it will influence your friends, especially the ones closest to you—your fellowship. You will find the strength and the support to become healthier together. And your influence will extend to all of your friends, and your friends' friends, and even their friends.

Friends helping friends. That's how you end the trend of obesity and disease. That's how you create a revolution. Are you ready? Let's go!

CHAPTER 12

CREATING A REVOLUTION

Never worry about numbers. Help one person at a time and always start with the person nearest you.[1]
— MOTHER THERESA

We are the Bibles the world is reading; we are the creeds the world is needing; we are the sermons the world is heeding.[2]
— BILLY GRAHAM

God has promised forgiveness to your repentance, but He has not promised tomorrow to your procrastination.[3]
— SAINT AUGUSTINE

In early November 2012, I received a call from my dad. I could immediately tell something was wrong. He was calling to make sure we were coming for Thanksgiving. He wanted to make sure he had everyone together because he was afraid it would be his last.

Dad had dealt with chronic pain for 17 years since a boating accident that had happened when he was working as a photographer for a large boat manufacturer. The accident left him with severe damage to his cervical column and permanent nerve damage. Prior to the accident, Dad had been training to compete in a senior power lifting competition. After the accident, unable to return to power lifting and dependent on narcotics to control the pain, he began a downward spiral into depression, diabetes and obesity. In November 2010, he suffered a bi-lateral hernia that would not be discovered until August of 2011 when he collapsed in his driveway. He was transported to an ER where they found and repaired the hernia. They also discovered that he was pre-diabetic, but nothing was done about that.

Not long after the surgery, dad began to suffer from extreme abdominal discomfort again. He saw specialist after specialist, but none of them could give him any answers. Dad's depression worsened. He had no answers for his abdominal pain, and he was starting to have chronic pain all over. He struggled to walk the 300 feet from his house to the barn and back without feeling exhausted and experiencing pain in his legs and feet. He couldn't even lie in bed with the sheets over him without pain.

His medications increased his appetite, so his weight soared up to 242 pounds and his body fat percentage to 42. Dad believed he was dying. The doctors and medications had no answers for him.

I wasn't ready to give up and lose my dad again, so I asked if he would be willing to do a cleanse with me. No promises . . . I just suggested that we do it together to see if it would help. My brother, Zach, and I bought him the Ultimate Reset® for Christmas, and I promised I would come up to Nashville to get him through the first week. On December 16, 2012, Dad was diagnosed with full-blown diabetes and advanced neuropathy, which is what was causing the pain in his legs and feet. On December 30, 2012, we began the Ultimate Reset together, along with his wife, Cate. That first week wasn't easy for him. That's why I was there. I wasn't going to let him give up. I knew if I could just get him through the first week, he could make it.

And he did.

Dad started feeling so much better that he joined the YMCA and started exercising again. He kept eating clean and completely reversed both the diabetes and neuropathy. His recovery was so rapid and so amazing that it floored his doctor, who said in 40 years of practicing medicine he had only ever seen one other person have that kind of recovery. Dad started volunteering at the local diabetes group at the Y because he wanted to help others. He still helps those he can and gets frustrated with the people who just want their medication so they can eat whatever they want. He now sees that mindset for the lie it truly is.

By the time we were all together again for the next Thanksgiving, Dad was down 78 pounds and had a 32-inch waist for the first time since he was in college. The best part was that he felt so much better. My dad got a new lease on life, and I get to have him around longer.

My kids also will get to enjoy more time with their granddad. For example, he was able to teach Reese how to use the tools in his wood shop, and Reese used that knowledge to build a Pinewood Derby car that smoked every other car in every race. He easily took the Pack, District, and Council championships. That was a proud multi-generational moment—a moment we may have missed had dad not turned his health around—had I not returned the favor and spoke truth into his life.

That's how we create a revolution—one life at a time. That's how all revolutions are born, with a small group of people passionate and committed to their cause. That's how God did it. He sent Jesus, who chose the disciples and poured His life into theirs. After His crucifixion, resurrection, and ascension, Jesus sent the Holy Spirit to empower those followers. They went out and "turned the world upside down" (Acts 17:6).

The Great Commission was not just for those early disciples; it is for us too. Jesus said, "I have been given all authority in heaven and on earth. Therefore, go and make disciples of all the nations, baptizing them in the name of the Father and the Son and the Holy Spirit. Teach these new disciples to obey all the commands I have given you. And be sure of this: I am with you always, even to the end of the age" (Matthew 28:18–20 NLT).

God's plan is for us to "Go and make disciples." We can't very well go if we can barely walk a flight of stairs. God's plan is for us to teach these new disciples all that He has commanded us, which, as Paul reminded us is all of Scripture (2 Timothy 3:16-17). So, part of what we are to instruct God's people on is His heart and design for our health. Taking care of our bodies is one of our spiritual disciplines.

Have I mentioned how faith and fitness are interwoven? Have I mentioned that I have led more people to Christ and done more ministry as a health coach than I did in full-time vocational ministry? I get to meet people from all backgrounds and walks of life and help them with a very real problem in their lives. I get to coach them through their transition into a healthier lifestyle. I get to walk with them on their first steps of that journey. I get to create relationships that will hopefully last a lifetime.

And through all of this, they get to hear about my great God and Savior. They get to hear about how much He loves them. They get to hear how He wants to make them complete—spirit, soul and body.

And I'm not alone. God is raising up an army of His sons and daughters to heal His people and tear down strongholds. This is not my message. It is not their message. It is *His* message. Ask God to speak to your heart. Answer the call. Join the revolution.

WHOEVER HAS EARS

Open war is upon us whether we would risk it or not. More than anything, I wish there was something I could say or do to help you see the reality of this war. It has been my constant prayer as I have written this book that God would give me the words because I know I am insufficient on my own. It troubles me that I may be misunderstood. But I am confident that God will speak to your heart. I pray that you will hear and receive His voice and take action.

Jesus often spoke in parables, simple little stories about earthly things that carry a huge spiritual meaning. Matthew, Mark, and Luke each record one that has come to be known as The Parable of the Sower (Matthew 13:1-23; Mark 4:1-20; Luke 18:1-15). In this story, Jesus revealed that there are four possible responses to the Word of God. We can reject it. We can accept until things get tough. We can miss it because of the distractions of the world. Or we can jump in with both feet for all it's worth.

At the end, Jesus said that whoever had ears to hear needed to listen. That's what is relevant for us—the truth that our response is based on our willingness to hear.

When the disciples ask Jesus to explain this parable to them, He said that seed represents God's Word, while the different soils each represent one of the four possible responses mentioned above. But it's all about the hearing.

Of course, Jesus wasn't talking about just physically hearing words. He was focusing on a deeper level of hearing—one that transforms the mind, engages the heart, and produces action. I pray that Jesus will say of you, as he did the disciples, "blessed are your eyes because they see, and your ears because they hear" (Matthew 13:16 NIV).

It's not enough to know what we should do. It's not even enough to want to do what is right. As Dallas Willard said in *The Spirit of the Disciplines: Understanding How God Changes Lives*:

> The general human failing is to want what is right and important, but at the same time not to commit to the kind of life that will produce the action we know to be right and the condition we want to enjoy. This is the feature of human character that explains why the road to hell is paved with good intentions. We intend what is right, but we avoid the life that would make it reality.[4]

Whoever has ears to hear, let them hear.

TIME TO CHOOSE

> *We must come to the Bible with the purpose of self-exposure consciously in mind.* I suspect not many people make more than a token stab in that direction. It's extremely hard work. It makes Bible study alternately convicting and reassuring, painful and soothing, puzzling and calming, and sometimes dull—but not for long if our purpose is to see ourselves better.[5]
> — Larry Crabb, *Inside Out*

It breaks my heart to know that some will refuse to do what is necessary to take control of their health. I know this from almost 10 years experience as a health coach. I know because James warned us to be doers of the word and not hearers only (James 1:22). I know this because Jesus told us that there are those who are not willing to hear.

It breaks my heart because I see people all around me living with the consequences of not doing whatever is necessary to be fully alive. As I have said before, we are all free to make our choices, but we are not free from their consequences. We have been warned, "Do not be deceived: God is not mocked, for whatever one sows, that will [they] also reap" (Galatians 6:7 ESV).

We are encouraged to choose life over death. There are some very sobering passages in Scripture—warnings that when we ignore the wisdom of God, He will leave us to our own devices. The Lord laments, "But my people did not listen to my voice; Israel would not submit to me. So I gave them over to their stubborn hearts, to follow their own counsels. Oh, that my people would listen to me, that Israel would walk in my ways! I would soon subdue their enemies and turn my hand against their foes" (Psalms 81:11–14 ESV).

We see this kind of warning throughout Scripture. We see Jesus weeping over Jerusalem, longing for His people to hear and understand and repent (Luke 19:41-44). We see the warnings to the churches in Revelation, especially the church at Laodicea (Revelation 3:14-22). God wants to heal us and give us a full life; but if we will not listen, understand and act, we have no one to blame but ourselves when the consequences of our actions come bearing down on us.

A few weeks ago at church, one of our campus ministers shared that he read a chapter in Proverbs every day. I took that as a challenge; so the next day, I read the first chapter of Proverbs. It contains both warning and promise. On one hand, if you listen and obey the voice of wisdom, you will live in peace. On the other hand, if you continue to bury your head in the sand, or walk in willful disobedience, ultimate disaster will overtake you like a storm.

The really sobering part is when it says:

"I called you so often, but you wouldn't come. I reached out to you, but you paid no attention. You ignored my advice and rejected the correction I offered. So I will laugh when you are in trouble! I will mock you when disaster overtakes you— when calamity overtakes you like a storm, when disaster engulfs you like a cyclone, and anguish and distress overwhelm you" (Proverbs 1:24-27 NLT).

Our lives depend on whether or not we heed the voice of wisdom. "Fools are destroyed by their own complacency. But all who listen to me will live in peace, untroubled by fear of harm" (Proverbs 1:30–33 NLT).

We are quick to point out these verses when it comes to someone else's sin, but aren't nearly as comfortable when it's applied to us. But it does apply to us, doesn't it? If someone smokes a pack of cigarettes a day and ends up with lung cancer, you would understand that they were reaping the consequences of their actions. If someone plays in traffic and gets hit by a car, you wouldn't be surprised. And if someone eats a diet of highly-processed foods loaded with sugar, fat, salt, artificial sweeteners and colors, chemicals, and GMOs then lays around on the couch every night, bad things will happen. They will end up with diabetes and heart disease, living out the last decade of their prematurely short life in pain. They are simply reaping the whirlwind.

Thank God, it doesn't end there. Each of God's warnings comes with a promise. As God told the Israelites, "If you will listen carefully to the voice of the LORD your God and do what is right in his sight, obeying his commands and keeping all his decrees, then I will not make you suffer any of the diseases I sent on the Egyptians; for I am the LORD who heals you" (Exodus 15:26 NLT). God's offer is life.

GETTING IT RIGHT

I remember walking through church one day with our kids. As we passed by the welcome area, we walked past a table full of donuts and pastries. Reese, who was 7 at the time, looked over at the table and said, "Mom, why do they have donuts at church? Don't they know donuts are bad for you?" Sam, on the other hand, who was 5, saw them and excitedly said, "Mommy, they have donuts at church! They must not be bad for you!"

Donuts are a touchy subject in church, especially when I mention that I don't think we should be serving them. The typical response is rolled eyes and something along the lines of, "Oh c'mon! You can't be serious. It's just a donut. Don't be such a killjoy." You're right. It is just a donut. But a donut is high fat and high sugar. That makes it addictive. It also makes it one of the worst possible things you can put in your body before you go into a worship service.

When you eat a donut, or any other high glycemic food (including bagels), a couple of things happen—very similar to the soda example in Chapter 8. First, your brain responds to sugar the same way it does to cocaine. It releases a surge of the feel-good brain chemicals dopamine and serotonin. That's what makes it addictive. And that's why you feel so good right after you eat it. So, you eat the donut and walk into the worship service and you feel amazing as you sing the worship songs. Meanwhile, your body releases insulin to absorb the excess glucose in your blood in an attempt to normalize your blood sugar. That leads to the infamous sugar crash when your blood sugar drops again because the insulin did its job. So you were on this amazing high, then you completely crash—and it's all you can do to stay awake right about the time the sermon starts.

You've just significantly crippled your ability to pay attention and learn. Brain fog sets in and by the time you head out the door you can hardly remember what was said. And, no, the coffee doesn't help, especially if you added sugar—or worse, sugar *and* cream—to it.

Let me take it a step further: You say it's just one donut, but would you offer just one drink to an alcoholic? Would you offer just one cigarette to someone who was struggling to quit smoking? So why would you offer one donut and tempt the diabetic and the sugar addict?

You might think that's a bit drastic, but is it?

It undermines the mission of the church. What if every follower of Christ was healthy and strong enough to serve in missions and ministries? What if we weren't having to spend so much time and money on doctors and medications for illnesses we could have prevented in the first place? What if we funneled those resources into the Kingdom?

Which takes me back to the beginning: What is the heart of God in all of this?

If this book has come across as a list of rules to follow, I sincerely apologize. This is not about rules. It is not about laying out a set of principles to be meticulously followed. This is not about being "religious" in how we eat and work out.

It is not about religion at all. It's about relationship.

You can do all of the right things, and still miss what matters most—a deep and growing relationship with God. Without that relationship, it doesn't matter what else you do because you will never be fully alive. No, the heart of this book is *not* to teach you to follow a set of rules. It is to teach you to walk with God. That's what we were created for, "to glorify God, and to enjoy Him forever"[6]—starting now.

John Eldredge put it like this:

> You might recall the old proverb: "Give a man a fish and you feed him for a day; teach a man to fish and you feed him for a lifetime." The same holds true here. Teach a man a rule and you help him solve a problem; teach a man to walk with God and you help him

solve the rest of his life. . . . Only by walking with God can we hope to find the path that leads to life. That is what it means to be a disciple. After all—aren't we 'followers of Christ?' Then by all means, let's actually follow him. Not ideas about him. Not just his principles. Him.[7]

And that's it. If we are walking with Him, we will submit to His will in every area of our lives—and He will sanctify us spirit, soul, and body. We will be transformed from glory to ever increasing glory. We will live fully alive!

"Now to Him who is able to [carry out His purpose and] do superabundantly more than all that we dare ask or think [infinitely beyond our greatest prayers, hopes, or dreams], according to His power that is at work within us, to Him be the glory in the church and in Christ Jesus throughout all generations forever and ever. Amen." (Ephesians 3:20-21 AMP)

NOTES

INTRODUCTION

[1] Irenaeus of Polycarp, quoted by John Eldredge in *Waking the Dead: The Glory of a Heart Fully Alive*, (Nashville: Thomas Nelson, 2006), Kindle Edition, 10.
[2] Oswald Chambers, *My Utmost For His Highest: An Updated Edition in Today's Language*, (Nashville, TN: Discovery House Publishers, 1992), December 5.

CHAPTER 1: WE ARE AT WAR

[1] J.R.R. Tolkien, *The Lord of the Rings: The Two Towers*, directed by Peter Jackson, 2002. USA: New Line Cinema, 2003 DVD.
[2] Ibid.
[3] T.D. Jakes on Twitter, https://twitter.com/BishopJakes/status/821688845972414464.
[4] Darren Hardy, *The Compound Effect*, (New York: Vanguard Press, 2011), Kindle Edition, 33.
[5] "Obesity Rates & Trends Overview," stateofobesity.org, http://stateofobesity.org/obesity-rates-trends-overview/
[6] "State Obesity Rates Could Skyrocket by 2030," USAToday.com, September 18, 2012. http://www.usatoday.com/story/news/nation/2012/09/19/state-obesity-rates-skyrocket/1576757/
[7] "The vast majority of American adults are overweight or obese, and weight is a growing problem among US children," Institute for Health Metrics and Evaluation, http://www.healthdata.org/news-release/vast-majority-american-adults-are-overweight-or-obese-and-weight-growing-problem-among
[8] "UN: Chronic Ailments More Deadly Than Infectious Diseases," CNNhealth.com, May 22, 2008. http://www.cnn.com/2008/HEALTH/05/22/world.death/
[9] Mark Hyman, M.D., *The Blood Sugar Solution 10-Day Detox Diet: Activate Your Body's Natural Ability to Burn Fat and Lose Weight Fast*, (New York: Little, Brown and Company, 2014), Kindle edition, 15.
[10] David Ludwig, M.D., "Children's Life Expectancy Being Cut Short by Obesity," *The New York Times*, March 17, 2005, http://www.nytimes.com/2005/03/17/health/childrens-life-expectancy-being-cut-short-by-obesity.html?_r=0
[11] Stephen Adams, "Obesity Killing Three Times as Many as Malnutrition," *The Telegraph*, December 13, 2012. http://www.telegraph.co.uk/news/health/news/9742960/Obesity-killing-three-times-as-many-as-malnutrition.html

[12] "Panel: Obesity is century's greatest public health threat," *USA Today*, http://usatoday30.usatoday.com/news/health/weightloss/2010-06-15-dietaryguidelines16_ST_N.htm

[13] Krista M. C. Cline, and Kenneth F. Ferraro. "Does Religion Increase the Prevalence and Incidence of Obesity in Adulthood?" *Journal for the Scientific Study of Religion* 45, no. 2 (2006): 269-81. http://www.jstor.org/stable/3838317.

[14] Wendy Ashley, "Obesity in the Body of Christ," *SBCLife*, http://www.sbclife.net/Articles/2007/01/sla8

[15] Matthew Feinstein, et al, "Incident Obesity and Cardiovascular Risk Factors Between Young Adulthood and Middle Age by Religious Involvement: The Coronary Artery Risk Development in Young Adults (CARDIA) Study." *Preventive Medicine* 54.2 (2012): 117–121. *PMC*. Web. March 12, 2017.

[16] Maria Paul, "Religious Young Adults Become Obese By Middle Age," March 23, 2011, http://www.northwestern.edu/newscenter/stories/2011/03/religious-young-adults-obese.html

[17] Scott Stoll, M.D., "Fat in Church," January 4, 2012, http://www.foxnews.com/opinion/2012/06/03/obesity-epidemic-in-america-churches.html

[18] Ibid.

[19] Ibid.

[20] Mercedes R. Carnethon, PhD; Peter John D. De Chavez, MS; Mary L. Biggs, PhD; et al, "Association of Weight Status With Mortality in Adults With Incident Diabetes," *JAMA*. 2012;308(6):581-590, http://jamanetwork.com/journals/jama/fullarticle/1309174.

[21] Rick Warren, "Secrets to Weight Loss with Pastor Rick Warren," *The Dr. Oz Show*, December 2, 2011, http://www.doctoroz.com/episode/million-dollar-you-how-lose-weight-and-win-million-dollars?video_id=1847884853001

[22] Dana Key and Eddie Degarmo, "Casual Christian," Copyright © 1985, Dkb Music (ASCAP) (adm. at CapitalCMGPublishing.com) All rights reserved. Used by permission.

[23] Kenneth D. Kochanek, M.A., Sherry L. Murphy, B.S., Jiaquan Xu, M.D., and Betzaida Tejada-Vera, M.S., "Deaths: Final Date for 2014," National Vital Statistics Report, CDC Division of Vital Statistics, Vol 65. No. 4, June 30, 2016, https://www.cdc.gov/nchs/data/nvsr/nvsr65/nvsr65_04.pdf

CHAPTER 2: KNOW YOUR ENEMY

[1] A.W. Tozer, "In the World But Not of It," *Tozer Devotional*, September 6, 2016, https://www.cmalliance.org/devotions/tozer?id=561

[2] Sun Tzu, Wikiquote, https://en.wikiquote.org/wiki/Sun_Tzu

[3] J.R.R. Tolkien, *The Lord of the Rings: The Fellowship of the Ring*, directed by Peter Jackson 2001. USA: New Line Cinema, 2002 DVD.

[4] *Plunket's Food Industry Market Research*, https://www.plunkettresearch.com/industries/food-beverage-grocery-market-research/

5 "Here's What the Average American Spends on Restaurants and Takeout," https://www.fool.com/retirement/2017/01/01/heres-what-the-average-american-spends-on-restaura.aspx

6 E. Martínez Steele, LG Baraldi, MLDC Louzada, et al, "Ultra-processed foods and added sugars in the US diet: evidence from a nationally representative cross-sectional study," *BMJ* Open 2016; 6:e009892. doi: 10.1136/bmjopen-2015-009892

7 Michael Pollan, *Food Rules* (New York: Penguin Books, 2009), xv.

8 Paul Zane Pilzer, The New Wellness Revolution, Second Edition (Hoboken, NJ: John Wiley & Sons, 2007), 19.

9 Pilzer, 20.

10. Hyman, *The Blood Sugar Solution*, 21-22.

11 "Conflicts of Interest as a Health Policy Problem: Industry Ties and Bias in Drug Approval," http://ethics.harvard.edu/conflicts-interest-health-policy-problem-industry-ties-and-bias-drug-approval

12. Walter C. Willett, M.D., Dr. P.H., *Eat, Drink, and Be Healthy: The Harvard Medical School Guide to Healthy Eating,* (New York: Free Press, 2005), 14.

13 Andrew Weil, M.D., "U.S. manages disease, not health," *CNN,* http://www.cnn.com/2013/03/08/opinion/weil-health-care/

14 *Escape Fire: The Fight to Rescue American Healthcare* (2012: Lionsgate Home Entertainment, 2013) DVD.

15 "Medical Definition of Iatrogenic," http://www.medicinenet.com/script/main/art.asp?articlekey=3886

16 Ronald Grisanti, D.C., D.A.B.C.O., D.A.C.B.N., M.S., "Iatrogenic Disease: The 3rd Most Fatal Disease in the USA," http://www.yourmedicaldetective.com/public/335.cfm

17 "Iatrogenesis," *Wikipedia,* https://en.wikipedia.org/wiki/Iatrogenesis

18 Donald W. Light, "New Prescription Drugs: A Major Health Risk With Few Offsetting Advantages," *Harvard University Blog,* June 27, 2014, http://ethics.harvard.edu/blog/new-prescription-drugs-major-health-risk-few-offsetting-advantages

19 *Thayer's Greek-English Lexicon of the New Testament,* paragraph 9640. Electronic edition.

20 *Strong's Greek Dictionary of the New Testament,* paragraph 1. Electronic edition.

21 Kenneth S. Wuest, *Galatians in the Greek New Testament,* http://www.chirpz.com/wp-content/uploads/downloads/2013/04/Galatians-GNT-by-Kenneth-Wuest.pdf

22 W.E. Vine, M. F. Unger, and W. White, *Vine's Complete Expository Dictionary of Old and New Testament Words,* (Nashville: Thomas Nelson, 1984), electronic edition.

23 Ibid.

24 J. Hampton Keathley, III, "25. Destruction of Commercial Babylon (Rev. 18:1-24)," *Studies in Revelation,* 2009. https://bible.org/seriespage/25-destruction-commercial-babylon-rev-181-24

[25] A.W. Tozer, "The Christians Greatest Enemy" excerpted from *Rut, Rot or Revival,*
https://www.truthforfree.com/html/article_christiansgreatestenemy.html

CHAPTER 3: FIGHT FOR YOUR LIFE

[1] *Gladiator*, directed by Ridley Scott (2000: DreamWorks Pictures). DVD.
[2] Michael Jordan,
https://www.brainyquote.com/quotes/quotes/m/michaeljor447185.html
[3]. Albert Barnes, *Barnes' Notes on the New Testament*, Accordance electronic ed. (Altamonte Springs, FL: OakTree Software, 2006), paragraph 18455.
[4] John Piper, "Olympic Spirituality Part 2,"
http://www.desiringgod.org/messages/olympic-spirituality-part-2
[5] *Gladiator*, directed by Ridley Scott (2000: DreamWorks Pictures). DVD.
[6] "Simon Sinek – Millenials in the Workplace,"
https://www.youtube.com/watch?v=5MC2X-LRbkE
[7] Jim Rohn, *Goodreads.com*, https://www.goodreads.com/quotes/905713-take-care-of-your-body-it-s-the-only-place-you
[8] John F. Kennedy, in *Physical Activity & Health: An Interactive Approach*, (April 19, 2011), 21. https://en.wikiquote.org/wiki/Body
[9] Oswald Chambers, *My Utmost For His Highest* (December 5)
[10] Roy E. Ciampa, Brian S. Rosner, *The First Letter to the Corinthians (The Pillar New Testament Commentary)* (Eerdmans Publishing, 2010-11-09), Kindle Edition, 251.
[11] Ibid., 252.
[12] Elton Trueblood, as quoted in *Leadership*, vol. 10. no. 3. Summer 1989, 60.
[13] *Gotta Serve Somebody*, 1979.
[14] Ciampa, 249.
[15] C. Edwards, *The Politics of Immorality in Ancient Rome* (Cambridge: Cambridge University Press, 1993), 188. Cf. Winter, Seek the Welfare of the City,174, who cites Dio Chrysostom as saying that brothel-keepers "drag their stock" to the "great festive occasions," cited in Ciampa, 249.
[16] Garland, D. E., *1 Corinthians (Baker Exegetical Commentary on the New Testament)*, (Grand Rapids: Baker, 2003). 474.
[17] Ibid., 239.

CHAPTER 4: THE HEART OF WORSHIP

[1] C.S. Lewis, quoted in "Great Quotes on Worship," *Experiencing Worship*, September 14, 2013, http://www.experiencingworship.com/worship-articles/general/2001-7-Great-Quotes-on.html
[2] James Allen, *As a Man Thinketh*, quoted at Goodreads.com, https://www.goodreads.com/quotes/57595-he-who-would-accomplish-little-need-sacrifice-little-he-who
[3] John Piper, *Desiring God: Meditations of a Christian Hedonist* (Portland, OR: Multnomah Press, 1986), 94.

[4] C.S. Lewis, *The Weight of Glory and Other Addresses,* (New York: Macmillan, 1949). PDF

[5] Piper, *Desiring God,* 94.

[6] Eldredge, John (2016-09-13). The Journey of Desire: Searching for the Life You've Always Dreamed Of (p. 135). Thomas Nelson. Kindle Edition.

[7] John Piper, *Present Your Bodies As a Living Sacrifice to God* (June 13, 2004), http://www.desiringgod.org/messages/present-your-bodies-as-a-living-sacrifice-to-god.

[8] *New Oxford American Dictionary,* (Oxford: Oxford University Press, 2016), Apple Dictionary.

[9] Jim Rohn, "Success is Everything," *Get Motivation,* http://www.getmotivation.com/jimrohn/jrsuccess_everything.html

[10] Reinhold Niebuhr, "The Serenity Prayer," Wikiquote, https://en.wikiquote.org/wiki/Reinhold_Niebuhr

[11] C.S. Lewis, *Mere Christianity* (New York: Touchstone, 1996), 169.

[12] Jerry Bridges, *The Pursuit of* Holiness, (Colorado Springs: Navpress. 1996), 93.

[13] "Talent," Online Etymology Dictionary, http://www.etymonline.com/index.php?term=talent

[14] Augustine of Hippo, Wikiquote, https://en.wikiquote.org/wiki/Augustine_of_Hippo

CHAPTER 5: STRENGTH AND BEAUTY

[1] John & Stasi Eldredge, *Captivating,* (Nashville: Thomas Nelson, 2010), 35.

[2] Augustine, "City of God," in *Nicene and Post Nicene Fathers*, ed., Philip Schaff, Series 1, Vol. 2 (Grand Rapids: Christian Classics Ethereal Library, 1999), PDF, 694.

[3] Lewis, *The Weight of Glory.*

[4] John Eldredge, *Wild at Heart,* (Nashville: Thomas Nelson, 2010), iBook edition, 16.

[5] Ibid., 17.

[6] C.S. Lewis, *The Lion, the Witch, and the Wardrobe,* (New York: HarperTrophy, 1978), 86.

[7] Eldredge, *Wild at Heart*, 20-21.

[8] Angela Thomas, *Do You Think I'm Beautiful? The Question Every Woman Asks,* (Nashville: Thomas Nelson, 2003), Kindle edition.

[9] Eldredge, *Captivating*, 35.

[10] John Piper, "How Pervasive and Practical Is the Beauty of God?," http://www.desiringgod.org/articles/how-pervasive-and-practical-is-the-beauty-of-god

[11] Eldredge, *Captivating*, 35.

[12] Eldredge, *Captivating*, 37.

[13] Lewis, *The Weight of Glory.*

[14] Carmen Wong Ulrich, *The Real Cost of Living: Making the Best Choices for You, Your Life, and Your Money*, (New York: A Perigee Book, 2011), Kindle edition.

[15] Alex Sorondo, "The Fountain of Youth in Ancient Greece," http://classroom.synonym.com/fountain-youth-ancient-greece-9599.html.
[16] Tony Horton via Twiter, https://twitter.com/Tony_Horton/status/306919772736614404

FINDING FREEDOM

[1] C.S. Lewis, The Voyage of the Dawn Treader, (New York: HarperTrophy, 1980), 115-117.
[2] Rick Warren, Daniel Amen and Mark Hyman, *The Daniel Plan: 40 Days to a Healthier Life*, (Grand Rapids: Zondervan, 2013), 32.

CHAPTER 6: THE FOUNDATION OF FAITH

[1] Stuart Townend, "How Deep The Father's Love For Us," Copyright © 1995, Thankyou Music (PRS) (adm. Worldwide at CapitalCMGPublishing.com excluding Europe which is adm. by Intergrity Music, part of the David C. Cook family. Songs@integritymusic.com) All rights reserved. Used by permission.
[2] http://quoteinvestigator.com/2013/01/10/watch-your-thoughts/

CHAPTER 7: THE PILLAR OF FOOD

[1] Dr. Ann Wigmore, Goodreads.com, https://www.goodreads.com/quotes/563016-the-food-you-eat-can-be-either-the-safest-and
[2] C.S. Lewis, *The Screwtape Letters*, (Harper Collins, Kindle edition, 2009), 44-45, 46.
[3] Lewis, *The Screwtape Letters,* 113-116.
[4] Gary Vaynerchuk, "Content is King, But Context is God," https://www.garyvaynerchuk.com/content-is-king-but-context-is-god/
[5] D.A. Carson, *Exegetical Fallacies* (Grand Rapids: Baker, 1996), Electronic Edition.
[6] David Grotto, RD, LDN, Elisa Zied, MS, RD, CDN, "The Standard American Diet and Its Relationship to the Health Status of Americans," *Nutrition in Clinical Practice*, Vol. 25, issue 6, 7 December 2010, 603-612.
[7] Heather Morgan, MS, NLC, "Ready to Ditch the Girdle?" *Muffin Top Makeover*, http://muffintopmakeover.com/2012/01/03/ready-to-ditch-the-girdle/
[8]. William C. Roberts, Quoted by Darin Olien, *SuperLife: The 5 Forces That Will Make You Healthy, Fit, and Eternally Awesome* (New York: Harper Collins, 2015), Kindle Edition, 132.
[9] Jordan S. Rubin, N.M.D., Ph.D., *The Maker's Diet*, (Lake Mary, FL: Siloam, 2004).
[10] Lorie Johnson, "Secrets to Longevity Revealed in Denomination's Lifestyle," *CBN News,*

http://www1.cbn.com/cbnnews/healthscience/2015/February/Secrets-to-Longevity-Revealed-in-Denominations-Lifestyle.

[11] "LONGEVITY HOT SPOTS - Highest Life Expectancy In The World?," http://www.worldlifeexpectancy.com/longevity-hot-spots

[12] Mary MacVean, "Why Loma Linda residents live longer than the rest of us: They treat the body like a temple," http://www.latimes.com/health/la-he-blue-zone-loma-linda-20150711-story.html

[13] J. Vernon McGee, *Leviticus I: The Law (Leviticus 1-14)*, (Nashville: Thomas Nelson, 1995), Kindle edition, 114.

[14] Samuel H. Kellogg, *The Expositor's Bible: The Book of Leviticus* (Kindle Locations 3787-3789).

[15] Kellogg, (Kindle Locations 3833-3836).

[16] Gordon J. Wenham. *The Book of Leviticus* (New International Commentary on the Old Testament) (Kindle Locations 2251-2252).

[17] McGee, 114.

[18] John Gill, "Commentary on Proverbs 23:2," *The New John Gill Exposition of the Entire Bible.* (Winterbourne, Ontario: Online Bible,1999), http://www.studylight.org/commentaries/geb/proverbs-23.html.

[19] Peter Rothschild, M.D., Ph.D., *The Art of Health*, as cited in Rubin, 34.

[20] Maurice Fishberg, M.D., "The Comparative Pathology of the Jews" *New York Medical Journal* 73 (1901), 540.

[21] Ibid.

[22] Robert Jastrow, *God and the Astronomers*, (New York: W. W. Norton, 1978) 116.

[23] McGee, 114.

[24] Kellogg, (Kindle Locations 3793-3798).

[25] McGee, 114.

[26] Kellogg, (Kindle Locations 3807-3814).

[27] Bulletin of the History of Medicine, Volume XXVII, September-October, 1953, Number 5, 444-450.

[28] Idid,, 445.

[29] Ibid., 450.

[30] "The Black Death – Jewish History," http://www.jewishhistory.org/the-black-death/

[31] Idid.

[32] Fishberg, 541.

[33] Kellogg, (Kindle Locations 3831-3832).

[34] John M. Scudder, M.D., Mosaic Laws of Hygiene, *The Eclectic Medical Journal*, Volume 47, Cincinnati, 1887, p. 133

[35] Gary Smalley, *Food and Love*, (Carol Stream, IL: Tyndale House Publishers, 2001).

CHAPTER 8: FOODOLOGY

[1] Hippocrates, "Hippocrates Quotes," Goodreads.com, https://www.goodreads.com/author/quotes/248774.Hippocrates

[2] Thomas Edison, "Thomas Edison on the 'Doctor of the Future,'" Snopes.com, January 25, 2015, http://www.snopes.com/quotes/futuredoctor.asp
[3] Heather Morgan, MS, NLC, "Ready to Ditch the Girdle?" http://muffintopmakeover.com/2012/01/03/ready-to-ditch-the-girdle/
[4] Darin Olien, *SuperLife: The 5 Forces That Will Make You Healthy, Fit, and Eternally Awesome* (HarperCollins. Kindle Edition, 2015), 8.
[5] Kenneth D. Kochanek, M.A., Sherry L. Murphy, B.S., Jiaquan Xu, M.D., and Betzaida Tejada-Vera, M.S., "Deaths: Final Data for 2014" *National Vital Statistics Report.* Vol. 65, No. 4, June 30, 2016, 5. https://www.cdc.gov/nchs/data/nvsr/nvsr65/nvsr65_04.pdf
[6] "Dr. Sanjay Gupta Reports: The Last Heart Attack," *CNN*, http://cnnpressroom.blogs.cnn.com/2011/08/02/'dr-sanjay-gupta-reports-the-last-heart-attack'---a-mission-possible/
[7] Ibid.
[8] Ibid
[9] Kochanek. 5.
[10] Hyman. 44
[11] "The Human Exposome Project," http://humanexposomeproject.com
[12] "NIH Human Microbiome Project," http://www.hmpdacc.org
[13] "Carotenoids," Oregon State University, Linus Pauling Institute, Micronutrient Infromation Center, http://lpi.oregonstate.edu/mic/dietary-factors/phytochemicals/carotenoids
[14] "An introduction to free radical biochemistry," https://www.ncbi.nlm.nih.gov/pubmed/8221017
[15] Josh Axe, "Fighting Free Radicals & Free Radical Damage," https://draxe.com/fighting-free-radical-damage/
[16] "Blood-brain barrier," *Wikipedia*, https://en.wikipedia.org/wiki/Blood–brain_barrier
[17]. Mercola, "The Secrets of Resveratrol's Health Benefits," http://articles.mercola.com/sites/articles/archive/2009/08/18/the-secrets-of-resveratrols-health-benefits.aspx
[18]. https://en.wikipedia.org/wiki/Sulforaphane
[19]. Olien, 13.
[20] Betty Miller, "The Wisdom of God, Proverbs 23:1-3," http://www.crossmap.com/devotionals/the-wisdom-of-god-proverbs-23-1-3-1331
[21] "Essential Fatty Acids," *Physicians Committee for Responsible Medicine*, http://www.pcrm.org/health/health-topics/essential-fatty-acids
[22] Stefanie Cassetto, "Enjoy Superfoods for Better Health," *The Daniel Plan*, http://www.danielplan.com/healthyhabits/supperfoodoverview/
[23] David Wolfe, *Superfoods: The Food and Medicine of the Future*, (Berkeley, California: North Atlantic Books, 2009), 1.
[24] Idib.
[25] Olien, 102.
[26] Wolfe, 5, 225.

[27] Dr. Mercola, "Bad News About Pesticides," http://articles.mercola.com/sites/articles/archive/2014/04/29/pesticide-exposure.aspx

[28] "Kids on the Frontline," *Pesticide Action Network North America*, 2016, http://www.panna.org/resources/kids-frontline.

[29] Kagan Owens, Jay Feldman, and John Kepner, "Wide Range of Diseases Linked to Pesticides," http://www.beyondpesticides.org/assets/media/documents/health/pid-database.pdf.

[30] Lori Altman, "9 Diseases Linked to Pesticides," *Natural Health 365*, June 13, 2016, http://www.naturalhealth365.com/pesticides-toxic-chemicals-1868-html.

[31] "EWG's 2017 Shopper's Guide to Pesticides in Produce™," *Environmental Working Group*, https://www.ewg.org/foodnews/summary.php

[32] "Coca-Cola Product Facts," 2017, http://www.coca-colaproductfacts.com/en/coca-cola-products/coca-cola/.

[33] Dr. Mark Hyman, "Why Calories Don't Matter," http://drhyman.com/blog/2014/04/10/calories-dont-matter/.

[34] Warren, 84.

[35] http://www.coca-colaproductfacts.com/en/coca-cola-products/coca-cola/

[36] Hyman, "Why Calories Don't Matter."

[37] Hyman, "Why Calories Don't Matter."

[38] . Hyman, 17.

[39] Hyman, *The Blood Sugar Solution*, 29.

[40] Ibid,, 35-36.

[41] "Sugar 101," *American Heart Association*, 11 October 2016, http://www.heart.org/HEARTORG/HealthyLiving/HealthyEating/Nutrition/Sugar-101_UCM_306024_Article.jsp#.WN7TJBjMzUY

[42] Pollan, 41.

[43] "'Corn Sugar' Makers Hope You'll Buy The New Name," *NPR*, http://www.npr.org/templates/story/story.php?storyId=129971532

[44] Dr. Mercola, "Are You or Your Family Eating Toxic Food Dyes?" http://articles.mercola.com/sites/articles/archive/2011/02/24/are-you-or-your-family-eating-toxic-food-dyes.aspx

[45] Susanna Kim, "11 Food Ingredients Banned Outside the U.S. That We Eat," *ABC News*, 26 June 2013, http://abcnews.go.com/Lifestyle/Food/11-foods-banned-us/story?id=19457237

[46] Sheela Prakash, RD, "9 Negative Effects of Sports Drinks," *The Daily* Meal, October 11, 2013, http://www.thedailymeal.com/9-negative-effects-sports-drinks/101113

[47] Ibid.

[48] Patrick J. Skerrett, "Trade sports drinks for water," *Harvard Health Blog*, July 30, 2012, http://www.health.harvard.edu/blog/trade-sports-drinks-for-water-201207305079

[49] Sara Ipatenco, "The Harmful Effect of Sodium Nitrite in Food," Livestrong.com, March 13, 2014, http://www.livestrong.com/article/416466-the-

[50] Dr. Josh Axe, "What Are Nitrates? Reasons to Avoid Nitrates + Better Alternatives," *DrAxe.com*, https://draxe.com/nitrates/

[51] Mercola, "BPA Is Fine if You Ignore Most Studies for It," March 25, 2105, http://articles.mercola.com/sites/articles/archive/2015/03/25/health-risks-bpa.aspx

[52] Ibid.

[53] Mercola, "MSG: Is This Silent Killer Lurking in Your Kitchen Cabinets," April 29, 2009, http://articles.mercola.com/sites/articles/archive/2009/04/21/msg-is-this-silent-killer-lurking-in-your-kitchen-cabinets.aspx

[54] George R. Schwartz, M.D., *In Bad Taste: The MSG Symptom Complex*, (Santa Fe, New Mexico: Health Press, 1999).

[56] Bridges, 22.

CHAPTER 9: THE PILLAR OF FITNESS

[1] John J. Ratey, MD, *Spark: The Revolutionary New Science of Exercise and the Brain*, (New York: Little, Brown and Company, 2008) 3.

[2] Jordan Metzl, *The Exercise Cure: A Doctor's All-Natural, No-Pill Prescription for Better Health and Longer Life* (Rodale Books, 2014), Kindle Edition, 12.

[3] Hippocrates, "Hippocrates Quotes," Goodreads.com, https://www.goodreads.com/author/quotes/248774.Hippocrates

[4] R. Laird Harris, Editor; Gleason L. Archer, Jr., Associate Editor; Bruce K. Waltke, Associate Editor, *Theological Wordbook of the Old Testament*, (Chicago: Moody Bible Institute, 1980), Electronic text hypertexted and prepared by OakTree Software, Inc., 2:661.

[5] John & Stasi Eldredge, *Captivating*, (Nashville: Thomas Nelson, 2010), 33.

[6] *BDB Abridged*, Based on *A Hebrew and English Lexicon of the Old Testament*, by F. Brown, S. R. Driver, and C. A. Briggs. Oxford: Clarendon Press, 1907. Digitized and abridged as a part of the Princeton Theological Seminary Hebrew Lexicon Project under the direction of Dr. J. M. Roberts. Used by permission. Electronic text corrected, formatted, and hypertexted by OakTree Software, Inc. This electronic adaptation ©2001 OakTree Software, Inc., paragraph 13462.

[7] Eldredge, *Captivating*, 33.

[8.] Barnes, paragraph 26450.

[9] D. R Bassett,, P. L. Schneider, and G. E Huntington, "Physical activity in an Old Order Amish community," *Medicine and Science in Sports and Exercise, 36*, 1, January 01, 2004, 79-85. http://citeseerx.ist.psu.edu/viewdoc/download?doi=10.1.1.327.1998&rep=rep1&type=pdf

[10] Bassett quoted in "Why the Amish Rarely Get Sick or get Cancer: Things You Can Learn From Them," *Living Traditionally,* November 26, 2014, http://livingtraditionally.com/amish-rarely-get-sick-things-can-learn/

[11] Bassett quoted in "Raise a barn, feel the burn: It's Amishize!" *The Baltimore Sun*, January 18, 2004, http://articles.baltimoresun.com/2004-01-18/entertainment/0401200461_1_amish-community-order-amish-amish-men

[12.] Ratey. 3-4.

[13.] Tedd Mitchell, M.D., Tim Church, M.D., Ph.D., and Martin Zucker, *Move Yourself: The Cooper Clinic Medical Director's Guide to All the Healing Benefits of Exercise (Even a Little!)*, (Hoboken, NJ: John Wiley & Sons, 2008), 5, 6.

[14.] Metzl, 12.

[15.] Ibid. 31.

[16.] Ibid. 4.

[17.] Ibid. 6.

[18] Daniel G. Amen, *Change Your Brain, Change Your Life (Revised and Expanded): The Breakthrough Program for Conquering Anxiety, Depression, Obsessiveness, Lack of Focus, Anger, and Memory Problems* (Kindle Locations 6321-6322). Potter/TenSpeed/Harmony. Kindle Edition.

[19.] Ratey 3.

[20] Ratey, 40.

[21] Ibid.

[22.] Ratey 45.

[23] Ratey, 10.

[24] Ratey, 223.

[25.] Mitchell 74.

[26] Ratey, 48.

[27] Ratey, 51.

[28] Ibid.

[29] Ratey, 45.

[30] Ratey, 245.

[31.] "Study: Exercise Has Long-Lasting Effect On Depression," *Duke Today*, September 22, 2000, https://today.duke.edu/2000/09/exercise922.html

[32.] Ratey 7.

[33.] Mitchell 70.

[34] Mitchell, 41.

[35] Ibid.

[36] Mitchell, 42-43.

[37] Mitchell, 44.

[38] Mitchell, 46.

[39] Mitchell, 54.

[40] Metzl, 50.

[41] Metzl, 147.

[42] Mitchell, 62.

[43] Mitchell, 61.

[44] Ibid.

[45] Mitchell, 63.

[46] Chuck Norris, quoted on the back cover of Mitchell, *Move Yourself*.

[47] David Garcia, Nate Feuerstein and Toby McKeehan, "Till The Day I Die," Copyright © 2015, Achtober Songs (BMI) Capitol CMG Paragon (BMI) Universal Music – Brentwood Benson Publ. (ASCAP) D Soul Music (ASCAP) (adm. at CapitalCMGpublishing.com) All rights reserved. Used by permission.

[48] Dave Ramsey, "Gazelle Intensity: Do You Have It?"

[49] Tony Horton, *Bring It! : The Revolutionary Fitness Plan for All Levels that Burns Fat, Builds Muscle, and Shreds Inches,* (New York: Rodale, 2011), 253.
[50] Ibid., 254.

CHAPTER 10: THE PILLAR OF FOCUS

[1] Bruce Lee, "Bruce Lee Quotes," http://www.bruceleequotes.org/%E2%80%8Ethe-successful-warrior-is-the-average-man-with-laser-like-focus/
[2] Zig Ziglar, *See You at the Top*, Twenty-Fifth Anniversary Edition, (Gretna, LA: Pelican Publishing Company, 2003), 166.
[3] Dan Diamond, "Just 8% of People Achieve Their New Year's Resolutions. Here's How They Do It," *Forbes*, Jan 1, 2013, https://www.forbes.com/sites/dandiamond/2013/01/01/just-8-of-people-achieve-their-new-years-resolutions-heres-how-they-did-it/#7d6f45f3596b
[4] *New Oxford American Dictionary.*
[5.] Wansink, B. & Sobal, J. (2007). "Mindless Eating: The 200 Daily Food Decisions We Overlook." *Environment and Behavior*, 39:1, 106-123.
[6] Steven Furtick, Sun Stand Still, (Colorado Springs: Multnomah Books, 2010), 7.
[7] Denis Waitley, *The Psychology of Winning in the 21st Century*, Audiobook, 2015.
[8] Darren Hardy, *The Compound Effect,* (New York: Vanguard Press, 2011), Kindle edition, 61.
[9] Ibid.
[10] Hardy, 63-64.
[11.] http://www.desiringgod.org/articles/the-distance-between-head-and-heart
[12.] John Eldredge, *Waking the Dead: The Glory of a Heart Fully Alive,* (Nashville: Thomas Nelson, 2006), Kindle Edition, 41-42.
[13] "Courage," *Online Etymology Dictionary,* http://www.etymonline.com/index.php?term=courage
[14] "Inveniam viam," http://en.wikipedia.org/wiki/Inveniam_viam
[15] Eldredge, Waking the Dead, 153.

CHAPTER 11: THE PILLAR OF FELLOWSHIP

[1] "The Lord of the Rings: The Fellowship of the Ring Official Trailer #2 - (2001) HD," *YouTube*, https://youtu.be/aStYWD25fAQ
[2] John Eldredge, *Waking the Dead: The Glory of a Heart Fully Alive,* (Nashville: Thomas Nelson, 2006), Kindle Edition, 183.
[3] J.R.R. Tolkien, *The Lord of the Rings: The Fellowship of the Ring*, directed by Peter Jackson 2001. USA: New Line Cinema, 2002 DVD.
[4.] John Eldredge, *Waking the Dead*, 186-188.
[5] Andrew Mason, "The 59 One Anothers of the Bible," http://www.smallgroupchurches.com/the-59-one-anothers-of-the-bible/

[6] William D. Mounce, *Basics of Biblical Greek: Second* Edition, (Grand Rapids: Zondervan, 2003), 342.

[7] Andy Stanley, quoted by Mark Howell, "The Primary Activity of the Early Church," November 13, 2013, http://www.markhowelllive.com/the-primary-activity-of-the-early-church/

[8] Nicholas A. Christakis, M.D., Ph.D., M.P.H., and James H. Fowler, Ph.D, "The Spread of Obesity in a Large Social Network over 32 Years," *The New England Journal of Medicine*, July 26, 2007, PDF, available at http://www.nejm.org/doi/pdf/10.1056/NEJMsa066082.

CHAPTER 12: CREATING A REVOLUTION

[1] Mother Theresa, "Mother Theresa Quotes," Goodreads.com, https://www.goodreads.com/quotes/112196-never-worry-about-numbers-help-one-person-at-a-time.

[2] Billy Graham, "Billy Graham Quotes," Goodreads.com, https://www.goodreads.com/quotes/306084-we-are-the-bibles-the-world-is-reading-we-are

[3] Augustine, "St. Augustine: God has promised forgiveness," http://www.orthodoxchurchquotes.com/2013/07/12/st-augustine-god-has-promised-forgiveness/

[4] Dallas Willard, *The Spirit of the Disciplines* (San Fransisco, CA" HarperCollins Publishers, 1991), p. 6.

[5] Dr. Larry Crabb, *Inside Out: With Bonus Content* (Navpress, 2012), Kindle edition, 178.

[6] "The Westminster Shorter Catechism," http://www.westminsterconfession.org/confessional-standards/the-westminster-shorter-catechism.php

[7] John Eldredge, *Waking the Dead: The Glory of a Heart Fully Alive*, (Nashville: Thomas Nelson, 2006), Kindle Edition, 96-97.

NOTES

ABOUT THE AUTHOR

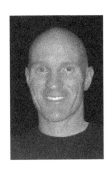 Deryl W. Duer has lived the message of this book. He is an acclaimed fitness expert, a Certified Personal Trainer (CPT) and Certified Health Coach (CHC). He's also a certified trainer in P90X Live, Insanity Live, and Turbokick. Deryl is a former law enforcement officer with 20 years of martial arts training. He graduated with honors from Liberty University and attended Southern Baptist Theological Seminary. Most importantly, Deryl is a husband and father of four.